Chart A

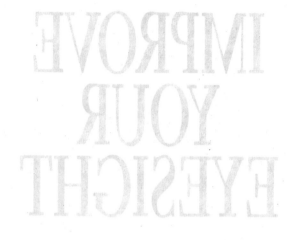

IMPROVE
YOUR
EYESIGHT

IMPROVE YOUR EYESIGHT

A Guide to the Bates Method for Better Eyesight without Glasses

Jonathan Barnes

SOUVENIR PRESS

The author and publishers are
grateful to Mrs Laura Huxley and
Chatto & Windus for permission to
reprint the extract from *The Art of
Seeing* by Aldous Huxley on p. 36.

First published in Australia by
Angus & Robertson Publishers
and in the United Kingdom by
Angus & Robertson (UK)

This edition first published 1999 by
Souvenir Press Ltd.,
43 Great Russell Street, London WC1B 3PA

Reprinted 1999, 2000 (3 times), 2001, 2003, 2004, 2006, 2008, 2011, 2014

ISBN 978 0 285 63508 1

Printed and bound in India by Replika Press Pvt Ltd

Contents

List of Figures

Preface

Besides wearing glasses or contact lenses, absolutely nothing, nothing whatever, can be done to alleviate errors of focusing in the human eye.

This, in the West, is the currently held orthodox belief to which, at one time, after a university training in biology, I fully subscribed. But now I know it to be wrong. I have proved to myself that it is not only possible, but simple, inexpensive, and above all completely safe to alleviate, not only errors of focusing, but also a number of other errors which degrade the performance of that most miraculous feat of biological engineering, the human visual system.

I no longer bother with glasses. I drive safely without them, visit the theatre and cinema, go bird-watching. My eyesight has been so much improved that I can perceive, for example, a ten-centimetre (four-inch) thick power cable at a range of three kilometres (nearly two miles).

Together with this improvement in focusing ability, startling enough on its own, I have found a remarkable improvement in the quality of my eyesight as a whole. It has a new vividness, richness, and greater stereoscopic depth. I am able to detect moving objects more quickly and follow them more accurately. The steam rising from my coffee cup is now seen to be composed of individual particles. Colours are clearer, softer, more detailed and vibrant. Short-sightedness is automatically corrected when using binoculars; at the age of 16, before I ever needed glasses, I bought the best binoculars I could afford, and thought them very good indeed. In recent years, though, I had begun to doubt my first opinion of them. Either that, or they had somehow deteriorated through use. In any event I was thinking of changing them for a yet more expensive pair. But now I find that the deterioration had nothing to do with the binoculars: it was entirely in my own eye. The image they deliver now is, if anything, better, more subtle, and more detailed than ever.

The method I used is not new. It was devised by a very remarkable and persistent man, Dr W. H. Bates, an ophthalmologist who practised in New York between 1885 and 1922. He published his method in 1919.

The Bates method, revised and updated since, has helped thousands of people, but such is the peculiar nature of optical defects, and such is the conservatism of the medical profession, that it has been generally ridiculed or ignored. As a result, millions of people are now wearing glasses and need not be. Worse: it is my belief that glasses (and contact lenses)* actually cause deterioration of the sight and may even be responsible for or contributory to certain forms of eye disease.

In these pages, though, we will be concerned not so much with eye disease as with the restoration of normal functioning to eyes which would otherwise be considered healthy. In practice that usually means overcoming errors of focusing; the other errors will disappear at the same time.

If you wear glasses you will probably have been diagnosed as suffering from at least one of these conditions:

1 **myopia,** or short-sightedness;
2 **hypermetropia,** or long-sightedness;
3 **presbyopia,** or "old-age" sight;
4 **astigmatism**.

All of these respond to the Bates method. In addition, people who have normal eyesight can often improve their vision far beyond the accepted standard of 6:6 (or 20:20, as was). In other words, someone who can read the bottom line of an optician's chart at a distance of 6 metres (20 feet) — the ordinary standard — may, after practising the Bates method, be able to read the same line at 8, 10 or 12 metres. (See Appendix A for the method of measuring visual acuity.)

* Unless a distinction is made, the term "glasses" in this book should be taken to include artificial lenses of any kind.

This sounds so far-fetched that I neither want nor expect you to take my word for it. All I ask of you is an open mind and the willingness to discover for yourself that the method works. If, soon after beginning its gentle and restful practices, you find that there has been an improvement in your vision, no matter how temporary or slight, then you too will have discovered that it *is* possible to alter "errors of focusing in the human eye". And when, some time later, you experience your first flash of perfect eyesight, when literally you glimpse the potential of the method, I doubt if anyone will be able to dissuade you from going on.

And if, finally, you are able to see as I can see today, then the pleasure I have derived from writing this book will have been multiplied, and I shall have gone some way towards repaying the debt of gratitude I owe to Dr Bates and his followers.

PART ONE

First
Questions

You are no doubt already wondering: "What is the Bates method, and if it is so marvellous why haven't I heard about it before?"

Briefly, the method is a way of re-educating the eyesight. Errors of refraction (that is, of focusing) are regarded as temporary abnormalities which, when exposed to the healing and self-regulatory powers of the body, can be reduced in severity or eliminated altogether.

As to why you haven't heard about it before, there are several reasons. The first and most important is the attitude of the medical profession. In our culture we have come to rely too heavily on the theoretical approach to medicine. No cure can be truly acceptable unless and until there is a theory to explain it. The theory accounting for refractive error is the work of the German scientist Hermann von Helmholtz (1821–94), whose contribution to the study of the nervous system still dominates modern thinking. Helmholtz's theory states that the eye accommodates (changes focus for far and near objects) by means of changes in the shape of the lens. If the lens or its muscle system is faulty, or if the eyeball is congenitally malformed, then refractive errors will arise. Although there is even now some controversy over the exact mechanism by which the lens changes its shape, orthodox science has never questioned the basic tenet of the Helmholtz theory: that it is the lens which is solely responsible for changing the focal length of the eye.

The theory is eminently reasonable. It seems to be borne out by the anatomy of the eye. Among older people, who progressively lose elasticity of the lens, refractive error is assumed to be an inevitable concomitant of the passing years, so much so that graphs have been drawn showing loss of accommodation with increasing age. Furthermore it is actually possible to see changes in the curvature of the lens: reflections in the front and back surfaces may be observed by using a small flashlight. These Purkinje images, as they are called, are taken as the next best thing to observing the act of accommodation in a cross-sectioned living eye. And, as further evidence in support of the Helmholtz theory, science would cite the apparent ease with which glasses correct optical errors.

Another serious obstacle to acceptance of the Bates method was the personality of W. H. Bates himself. Having found empirically that the Helmholtz theory was lacking, he was far too quick to formulate a rival theory. Bates's proposal was that the eye accommodates, not by a change in the shape of the lens, but by a change in the shape of the eyeball itself, this change being brought about by the six extrinsic muscles which control the movement of the eye in its socket. Such an idea was rejected as nonsense, the more so when Bates adduced less-than-convincing evidence in some of his scientific papers dealing with accommodation in animals. From then on he became a subject of ridicule and professional hostility. His insights into the psychology of vision were ignored, as were the successes he achieved in his consulting room. These successes convinced him he was right and his colleagues wrong; he became more and more exasperated, and the dogmatic tone of his *Perfect Sight Without Glasses** verges, in places, on the aggressive. This did little to win over his critics.

The Bates method was served no better by some of the people who set themselves up as teachers. For every conscientious teacher of the method there were several who understood nothing whatever about it and saw in it only a means of exploiting the desperate patients whom orthodoxy had failed. In consequence, any suggestion that there might be something in visual re-education

*New York, 1919. Since reissued, in many editions, as *Better Eyesight Without Glasses* (for example, Souvenir Press, 1977; Granada Publishing, 1979).

is now dismissed as outright quackery.

This attitude of the ophthalmic profession has perhaps, in part, consciously or otherwise, been influenced by another consideration. Although by no means all members of the profession profit from the trade in glasses, there is no question but that there is a huge vested interest in the correctness of the Helmholtz theory.

Yet another obstacle stands in the way of the Bates method. Results are usually slow in coming and require of the student a good deal of application, even faith. It is so easy to go for the instant solution that few people give the method a fair chance. The person who has improved his or her vision is such a rarity that few opticians will have encountered any evidence that the method works. Those cases that have come to light have certainly been explained as examples of anomalous but spontaneous improvement which would have happened anyway.

The final obstacle to acceptance of the method is the curious nature of refractive errors and the perpetuating effect that glasses have on them. Glasses tend to fix and make permanent errors that would otherwise, in time, correct themselves. The longer glasses are worn, the more intransigent the errors become, and the less believable it becomes that they could ever be cured.

And yet, despite all these difficulties, the method persists. It enjoyed special popularity in the 1930s and 1940s, particularly after its enthusiastic endorsement by the writer Aldous Huxley, whose book on the method, *The Art of Seeing* (Chatto & Windus, 1943), has rarely been out of print since. There have been other books too, of varying quality. In one of the better ones, published in 1957, the Bates teacher C. A. Hackett analyses the results of 10 years' work in which she treated 2180 cases of refractive error. Of these, over 75 per cent achieved lasting improvement, of whom about 45 per cent (over a third of all students) were able to do without their glasses entirely.

Besides the thousands of people who have derived benefit from teaching, there are presumably many who have achieved some success working alone. As Huxley points out, a book of instruction is no substitute for a good teacher, but in the absence of a teacher a book of instruction is better than nothing. It is my hope that I have presented in the following chapters an exposition which is clear, understandable, and designed to bring the wonderful benefits of the Bates method to all who care about their eyesight and are dissatisfied with present forms of treatment. It is also my hope — even conviction — that future generations will regard the wholesale dispensing of glasses as yet another pitiable example of a misguided fashion in medicine, as quaint as wholesale bloodletting or trepanning, and almost as barbarous.

The Visual Process

To succeed with the Bates method no knowledge of anatomy or the psychology of vision is necessary. All that is needed is to follow the instructions in Part Two, and you may prefer to skip this and the next two chapters for the time being. However, even a slight acquaintance with the visual process will let you evaluate the reasoning behind the instructions and this in turn is likely to help your progress, for you will see that the method is as logical as it is mild. Understanding this will also, to a certain extent, prepare you for the very considerable astonishment of discovering for yourself that the method works.

The anatomy of the eye

Vision, of course, is the sense that animals have evolved using light to provide information about their surroundings. The simplest animals of all are, like plants, sensitive only to light itself. With increasing complexity, animals become capable of discerning contrast, movement, images, colour, and stereo depth.

Compared with that of the other senses, the potentiality of vision is very great, for it is capable of yielding detailed and highly specific information at a distance as well as near to. This is of profound importance for survival; among those animals whose way of life demands good vision, the evolution of the eye has reached incredible levels of development.

6

The eye of man is not the most structurally complex in the animal kingdom, but it is certainly one of the most advanced, serving a brain which is the most sophisticated creation evolution has yet produced. The quality of this computer is matched by the quality of its major input devices for external stimuli—the ears and the eyes.

In structure, the human eye is a typical vertebrate eye, of a pattern common to all mammals. It is a hollow sphere (actually a spheroid) filled with fluid under slight pressure. This pressure maintains the shape of the sphere.

The eye may be thought of as being divided into two compartments, front and rear, by the **lens,** an elastic, convex body about eight millimetres across. A perfectly clear fluid, the **aqueous,** fills the front compartment, while the larger rear compartment is filled by the more gelatinous **vitreous,** the third component of the **optical media** — the transparent contents of the sphere through which light must pass.

In anatomical terms, the sphere itself is made up of three distinct layers. These are the **sclera,** the **uvea** and the **retina.**

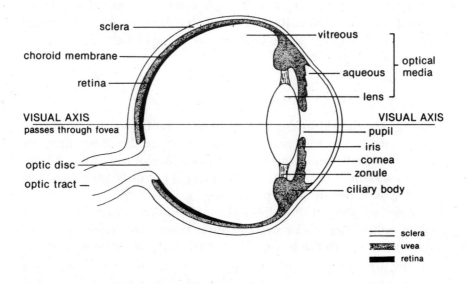

Figure 1. Horizontal section of the eye, showing terms mentioned in the text

The sclera is the outermost layer, the "white" of the eye, an extremely tough, fibrous sheath which protects the delicate structures within. At the front of the eye the sclera is modified into the **cornea,** a transparent, dome-shaped window which allows light to enter the eye.

The uvea consists of three parts: the **iris,** the **ciliary body,** and the **choroid membrane.** The iris lies just behind the cornea and is a muscular ring whose contractions can alter the size of the **pupil,** the aperture at its centre through which light gains access to the interior of the eye. The iris contains the pigment (brown, green, and so on) which gives the eye its "colour". Having passed through the pupil, light now passes through the lens, which is attached round its edge by a ligamentous membrane, the **zonule,** to the muscles of the ciliary body. Movements of these muscles alter the convexity of the lens, changing its focal length. The third and final part of the uvea is the choroid membrane. This is the network of blood-vessels lining much of the sclera, and provides the principal blood-supply for the inside of the eyeball.

The innermost layer of the eye is the retina, an exceedingly complex and delicate membrane of nerve-cells which includes the all-important **photoreceptors.** The photoreceptors are of two types, the **rods** and the **cones.** Rods are sensitive to dim light and register only shades of grey, while cones work in good light and are the source of colour vision.

Organisation of the retina

During the development of the human embryo, the forebrain bulges into buds which are destined to become the optic cups; the retina is actually an outgrowth of the surface of the brain, a kind of outpost where the visual information is not only generated but also receives preliminary processing.

There are some 130 million photoreceptors in each retina but only a million nerve fibres in the **optic tract** — the "cable" running from the retina to the brain. Thus each fibre must be shared, on average, by about 130 photoreceptors. Part of the work of the retina is to achieve this sharing without loss of picture quality. This feat is performed in the layers of specialised cells found between the photoreceptors and the nerve fibres. It is assisted by the way the photoreceptors are distributed throughout the retina.

The outer edges of the retina contain relatively few photoreceptors, mostly rods, and provide vision which may be compared to that of primitive animals. At the very periphery of the retina, indeed, there is no conscious vision at all, merely an awareness of movement and contrast. When you see something "in the corner of your eye" and automatically turn to see it better, you are responding to signals generated in this portion of the retina.

Further in towards the centre, the photoreceptors become more densely packed and the ratio of cones to rods increases. Occupying the centre is a region about 5.5 millimetres across, the **macula lutea** (usually abbreviated to "macula"). Towards the centre of the macula is a shallow depression called the **fovea centralis** or simply "fovea". The fovea is about 1.9 millimetres in diameter; at its centre, lying precisely on the **visual axis,** is an area only 0.35 millimetres across, the **foveola.**

In the fovea and foveola there are no rods, only cones, packed together so tightly that they look like rods. The cones reach their highest density in the foveola: the smallest cones here are less than one thousandth of a millimetre in effective diameter.

Throughout the retina as a whole, rods outnumber cones by about 18:1. It is the cones that are responsible for delivering precisely detailed vision. The importance of the cones is reflected in the generosity with which they are supplied with connections to the optic tract. Some of the cones in the foveola have exclusive use of a single nerve fibre. (In passing it is interesting to note that foveae, although found in certain fishes, lizards, and particularly in birds, do not occur in the lower mammals. Among mammals they appear only with the primates; the eye of the chimpanzee is remarkably similar to our own. Man's highly developed fovea, with the sharp sight it provides both at a distance and near to, has been one of the chief assets in his career as first a hunter, then a farmer, and now a technologist.)

The photoreceptors contain pigments which are bleached by exposure to light. This chemical change is converted into the electrical stimulus which then passes along the nerve to the brain. Once bleached, the pigments in any given photoreceptor take a little while to be replaced. Exposure to a very bright light will completely bleach a whole area of the retina and for a time its sensitivity will be impaired. This is the reason for the familiar after-images experienced after looking at anything very bright.

The muscles of the eye

Selection and control of the image falling on the retina is carried out by three muscle systems, two located inside the eyeball itself and the third outside.

The first of these systems is the iris. As has already been said, the iris is a muscular ring whose central aperture, the pupil, may be varied in size. As any photographer knows, to get the best from his film he must vary the aperture according to the prevailing light intensity. Controlling the amount of light entering the eye, though, is not the primary function of the iris, for, while the area of the pupil changes over a ratio of only about 16:1, the range of light intensities in which the eye works varies over a ratio of at least 1,000,000:1. The main function of the iris is probably to restrict the incoming light to the macula, except at times (such as dawn or dusk) when maximum sensitivity is needed. The pupil also contracts for near vision, "stopping down" the "camera" of the eye so that depth of focus is enhanced.

The pupil opens and closes automatically in response to the amount of light falling on the retina. In other words, there is feedback from the retina to the iris.

This idea of feedback is encountered several times in the study of vision. It is important in accommodation—the process in which the eye adjusts itself to focus on near or far objects. The feedback in accommodation comes from the part of the brain where perception takes place; if the image is out of focus, orders will automatically be sent to readjust the focusing mechanism.

Now we come to the central controversy of the Bates method: the means whereby accommodation is achieved. The currently accepted belief is that accommodation is attained solely through the action of the second internal muscle system of the eye, the ciliary body.

In this chapter the orthodox theory will be described, although even here there is dispute and uncertainty among ophthalmologists about the exact mode of action of the ciliary muscle and its nerve supply.

For distance vision the lens needs to be relatively flat, but to bring the converging rays from a near object into sharp focus, the lens must become more convex. (More about this is explained at the beginning of the next chapter.) The lens consists of a soft central filling enclosed by an elastic capsule. The wall of the capsule is thinner in some places than others, and its natural tendency is to bulge into a convex shape. Unless tension is applied to the capsule by way of the zonule, therefore, the soft filling will tend to form into a convex shape and so decrease the focal length of the lens.

Looking at Figure 1, it would seem evident that, because the more convex shape is the natural resting state of the lens, an effort has to be made only when distance vision is needed. Surprisingly, however, the opposite is the case. The lens is kept under permanent tension by the zonule, so that the usual shape is flattened and suitable for distance vision. When near vision is required, the ciliary muscle contracts, pulling the ciliary body forward. The diameter of the ciliary body (remember it is shaped like a ring) is thus reduced, tension in the zonule eases, and the capsule and with it the substance of the lens assumes a more convex shape.

More will be said about accommodation later; for the present, we will go back to our consideration of the three muscle systems of the eye.

The third of these systems consists of the six extrinsic muscles which control the movement of each eye in its orbit. The extrinsic muscles are arranged in three pairs, attached to the sclera and working together in such a way that the eye can be turned in various directions.

Most muscles of the body contain one of two types of fibre. Muscles under conscious control (for example, the muscles of the hand) contain **striped fibres,** but those associated with involuntary functions (such as digestion) contain **smooth** tissue. The extrinsic muscles of the eye, however, contain a unique mixture of both types. As we shall see next, the extrinsic muscles perform some functions which are automatic and others which are under the control of the will.

Eye movements

Our eyes are supremely well adapted to binocular vision—the rather unusual arrangement whereby both eyes share much the same field of view and, by giving two slightly different images, enable the brain to deduce information about depth. The eyes thus work in unison, as a dual organ, and their extrinsic muscles are perhaps the most delicate and sensitive to be found anywhere in the body.

The extrinsic muscles have at least four functions, which may be summed up as follows:

1 controlling the visual axes;
2 tracking;
3 searching;
4 scanning.

If you look across the room and then refocus on a finger held about 30 centimetres (12 inches) from your nose, you will notice that your eyes have become slightly "crossed": the two visual axes, instead of being virtually parallel, now converge on your finger. In this way both foveae are brought to bear on a single point.

For successful binocular vision, control of the visual axes must be very precise, and this control must of course also be maintained while the eyes are in motion.

The difference between the next two functions, tracking and searching, may be demonstrated quite simply. If you ask someone to follow a moving object (say your finger) with his eyes, you will notice that the eyes swivel smoothly in their sockets. If however you then ask the subject to perform the same eye movements on his own, without your finger to watch, his eyes will not move smoothly, but in a series of jerks.

Tracking, then, is quite different from searching. When tracking a moving target, a gunner must "lead the target" by aiming slightly ahead of it, the size of the lead being determined in part by the velocity and trajectory of the target and its distance from the gun. A practised shot uses his brain to perform the necessary computation almost instantaneously. It has been discovered that, while tracking, the eye must also lead the target. The eye anticipates the direction of movement by about six milliseconds (six thousandths of a second). The implications of this discovery are very remarkable indeed.

One might be forgiven for assuming that movements of the eyes are controlled, like muscle movements elsewhere in the body, by the brain. And in part, this assumption is correct. The commands directing the eyes to any part of the visual field arise in the brain; but what about the commands which enable the eyes to follow a moving object? The time required for the act of perception—for the light to stimulate the photoreceptors, for the nerve pulses to reach the brain, and for the brain to make sense of the signal — is in the order of 135 milliseconds. This delay alone, without even counting the time required for a return message from brain to eye muscles, is far too great to allow a "leading time" of only six milliseconds. If the commands came from the brain, the eyes would always be behind: they would never be able to focus on a flying bird or a moving tennis ball. Thus the guidance system that controls tracking cannot be located in the brain. It must be in the eye itself, almost certainly in the retina. We have already seen that the retina is in origin part of the surface of the brain. Besides the photoreceptors and their immediately associated cells, there are in the retina millions of other nerve-cells, very like those found in the brain itself, whose functions are still an almost total mystery.

The third type of eye movement, searching, has certain features in common with the fourth, scanning. As the second of our experiments showed, the eye searches the visual field by means of a series of jerks. Once something catches the attention, the jerks, or **saccades,** become smaller and are restricted to the region of the object being observed. Using an apparatus consisting of a minute mirror attached to a contact lens, researchers can trace these saccadic movements on photosensitive paper. When the subject is asked to fix his eyes on a single point, the tracings reveal that his gaze, while returning again and again to the point, wanders involuntarily over the surrounding area.

Because we see clearly only with the central portion of the retina, saccadic movement is necessary for exploration of the visual field. But its involuntary characteristcs are very like those of the fourth type of eye movement, a continuous, high-frequency tremor which here is called "scanning" — for reasons which will be apparent later.

Scanning is essential to vision. If, instead of a mirror, a miniature projector is attached to the contact lens, stabilising the image on the retina, vision rapidly fades. The subject sees the visual field becoming blurred and grey. Finally even the grey fades and is replaced by blackness. Then something unexpected happens. We are reminded that the brain is involved in vision as well as the eyes: from the blackness there emerge, in stately and inexplicable succession, one replacing another, ghostlike fragments of the original image.

Making sense of the signals

If vision can be likened to an end product whose raw material is light, the eye is no more than a supplier of crude and part-finished work to the main factory — the brain.

As we have already seen, a limited amount of preliminary processing of the raw visual data takes place in the retina, in two layers of cells called respectively the **bipolar cells** and the **ganglion cells.** To each bipolar cell are connected many individual photoreceptors, while, in turn, each photoreceptor is connected to a number of other bipolar cells. In a similar way, the bipolar cells are interconnected to the ganglion cells.

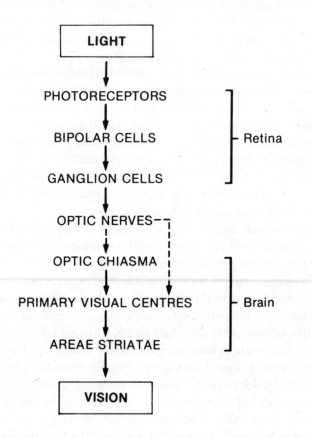

Figure 2: The pathway of information from retina to brain

From the ganglion cells, the electrical impulses leave the retina and are conducted along the optic tract towards the brain. The brain is divided into two hemispheres, left and right. Signals from the left-hand side of the left retina are conducted into the left hemisphere, but signals from the right-hand side of the left retina cross over into the right hemisphere. There is a similar cross-over from the left-hand side of the right retina. Thus the left hemisphere receives signals from the left-hand sides of both retinas and the right hemisphere receives signals from the right-hand sides. The point at which the pathways cross is called the **optic chiasma.** The signals next arrive at the **primary visual centre,** one in either hemisphere, where they are further processed before being sent on to the **area striata,** which is the region of the cerebral cortex devoted to vision.

The process of human perception is so intricate that only in recent decades has anything of value been learned about it. Attempts to equip machines with even rudimentary vision have increased our respect for the technical achievement of biological perception — and perception in man is almost certainly the most complex to be found in the living world. As for the way the area striata interacts with the rest of the cerebral cortex and, even more mysterious and fascinating, the way the cortex interacts with deeper regions of the brain, science has as yet uncovered virtually nothing.

The route of the nerve signals from retina to brain is summarised in Figure 2. In neurophysiological terms, analysis of the signals in the retina and also in the primary visual centre takes place by means of inhibition/excitation fields. The net result is that the area striata is fed with a coded version of the original image. The code is presented in terms of straight lines, movement, and colour.

Any image, however complex, can be resolved into a number of straight lines, however tiny those lines might be. A circle, for instance, can be thought of as an infinitely large number of very short straight lines, each one aligned with its neighbours at a constant and very precise angle. (Owners of home computers who know a program for generating polygons will be familiar with this idea: once the number of sides of the polygon reaches 50 or so, the computer in effect draws a circle on the screen. In human vision, the number of sides of the polygon has to be vastly greater before a smooth circle is perceived, but the principle is the same.)

The incoming code classifies the straight lines according to whether they are "edges", "strips", or "slits". It also classifies the movement, if any, of the image into its component directions. The area striata, by reading the code, translates it into a language of fantastic complexity — the language of vision.

The cerebral cortex, in which the area striata is found, is that part of the brain which, in man, is the seat of sensory perception, feelings, imagination, memory, thought, and indeed of personality itself. Although each area of the cortex is dedicated to one special function — such as hearing, word understanding, taste, vision, and so on — the different areas are interconnected by means of association fibres. This means in practice that our sensory perception, imagination, and so on, form an integrated and unified whole in which all parts of the cerebral cortex play a part.

Once a block of incoming code has been read, the information from either area striata — one dealing with the left-hand portion and the other with the right-hand portion of the original image — is recombined.

Studies of the psychology of vision have shown that, in order to understand the image being received by the eyes, the brain relies heavily on two associated functions of the cerebral cortex, imagination and memory. Seeing is an acquired skill as well as an innate one. Besides being a skill, it is also an art. In a real sense it is a creative process, like so many of the other functions of the cerebral cortex. Our past experience of the world is crucial to our present understanding of it. We learn certain rules (for example, that human beings, houses, trees, and so on tend to be of a certain size) and use them when trying to interpret an unfamiliar image. To demonstrate this, one has only to look at the well known optical illusion shown in Figure 3. Our experience of the world — and of stylised representations of it on paper — is such that we understand and accept the rules of perspective. Looking at the two sloping lines, we automatically assume that the rules of perspective are being invoked by the figure. It follows that the upper of the two horizontal lines must be farther away than the lower one. Therefore, the brain concludes, the upper line must be longer than the lower one, even though both are, of course, exactly the same length.

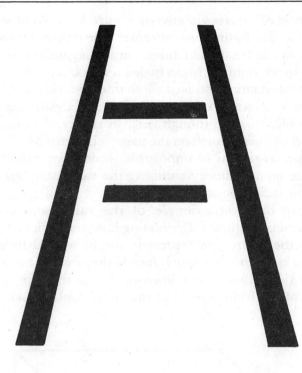

Figure 3: The Ponzo Illusion

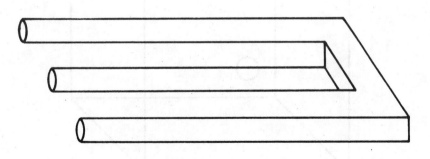

Figure 4: An impossible object

Another set of rules is violated by Figure 4. Looking at the left-hand end of the figure, we interpret the image received as a representation of the tips of three parallel cylinders. But as the eye travels to the right the brain makes a new interpretation, based on the new information received. Both interpretations are "correct", but each is mutually exclusive, and so the figure becomes an impossible object, even though it is, in reality, no more than a harmless set of lines printed on the page. The artist M. C. Escher's famous representations of impossible scenes—waterfalls flowing uphill, little men endlessly climbing the same staircase, and so on—rely on this technique.

A slightly different example of the same sort of idea is demonstrated by Figure 5. Depending how you look at it (literally speaking), the figure can represent one of several things. It is obviously a cube, but on which face is the circle? One answer is to say that the cube is tilted downwards and that the circle is in the centre of the front face—but the circle could equally well be

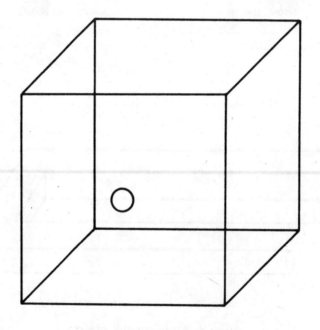

Figure 5: The Necker Cube

in the lower left corner of the rear face. Two further possibilities are presented if we regard the cube as being tilted upwards instead. Or again, the circle might be a sphere floating *inside* the cube, or some way behind or in front of it. Every solution is "correct" in perceptual terms; none is better than the others. The brain, however, insists that only one can be right, for this is how it perceives the world, choosing the best and most likely interpretation of the available data — the best guess. In this case the brain is unable to arrive at a decision and so the cube or the circle/sphere appears to jump back and forth according to the interpretation currently being entertained.

The visual process is, then, a function not only of the eyes and the immediately associated area of the brain, but of the cerebral cortex as a whole. Vision is a matter of memory and imagination as well as light. This will be understood immediately by anyone who has ever been fooled by one of those magazine pictures of familiar objects photographed from an unfamiliar angle, or who, in a contemplative moment, has ever seen faces in the fire. Our perceptual habits and beliefs are deeply influenced by our past experience, by our upbringing and background, and by the dictates of our personality. The way we look at the world is not only a unique expression of those habits: at the same time it confirms them and tends to make them more deeply ingrained.

Without going into the philosophical ideas raised by such a thought, we can say that there is a genuine biological basis for prejudice, for "pigeonholing", and for a variety of other practices which do no one any good. One unexpected and exciting by-product of visual retraining by the Bates method is a change of outlook for the better, accompanied by a steadily increasing sense of integration with the world at large.

THREE

Visual Defects

In a process as intricate as vision, it is not surprising that faults can and do often arise. This chapter will describe the commonest faults and try to relate each one to the point at which the visual process is going astray. It must not be forgotten, though, that vision is an integrated process and a fault in one area can often cause, or be caused by, a fault in another.

The visual defects discussed here are those from which the vast majority of people who wear glasses are suffering. The Bates method as usually practised, and as presented in this book, is concerned principally with the treatment of refractive error. But that is not to say that it cannot be of value to sufferers from other sorts of eye troubles. Because vision is an integrated process, a course of Bates training will benefit not only the eye's ability to focus, but also the health of the entire visual system. Minor infections and such irregularities as tics or mild squints often disappear within a few weeks of beginning the training. More serious conditions are also said to respond favourably, but by the time a case of cataract, for example, has advanced far enough for it to have been positively diagnosed, the Bates method can promise no more than a possible slowing of the progress of the condition. Rare cases, some quoted by Bates himself, of people with severe problems have achieved extraordinary results, but the method **must under no circumstances be regarded as a miracle cure for serious disease.** Cruel and unscrupulous claims to the contrary have done more than anything else to damage the prospects of the Bates method ever being properly investigated by the medical profession.

If you have a serious eye complaint you should think of the method as no more than an adjunct to the treatment you are already receiving. At worst, it can do no harm; at best, it might help you to a lesser or greater degree.

Errors of refraction

These are visual faults caused, usually, by defects in the cornea, lens, and in the shape of the eyeball itself. Before proceeding further, though, it might be as well to define exactly what is meant by "refraction".

Refraction is the deflection of light as it passes from one medium into another. The apparent bending of a stick dipped into water is due to the differing refractive powers of air and water; light is similarly refracted when it passes from air into glass (Figure 6).

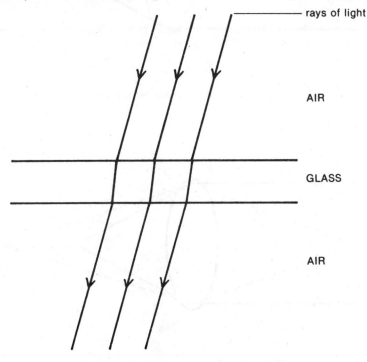

Figure 6: The principle of refraction

If the glass is curved, as in a lens, the nature of the refraction is changed (Figure 7). Now the rays of light, instead of continuing to travel onwards in parallel, are brought to a point—the focal point. It is at the focal point that a screen must be placed for a crisp image to be observed.

Figures 6 and 7 show the refraction of light from distant objects: that is, light whose rays are travelling, for all practical purposes, in parallel. Figure 8 shows what happens to the focal point when the lens receives the more divergent rays from a nearby object (dotted lines).

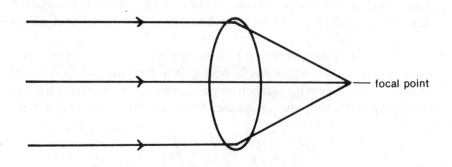

focal point

Figure 7: Refraction by a lens

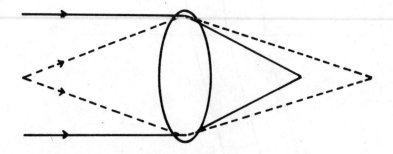

Figure 8: Refraction of light from near and far objects

If the lens is of a fixed shape, like a glass lens, the screen must be moved backwards to receive a crisp image of the nearby object, or else the lens itself must be moved. This is the method of focusing adopted in such man-made instruments as the optical microscope and the simple telescope.

Another way of changing the focus is to alter the shape of the lens. The more convex the lens, the greater its refractive power, and the greater its ability to focus light from nearby objects. This technique is used in the human eye.

Refraction in the eye is carried out not only by the lens, but also, and more importantly, by the cornea, which is strongly curved in cross-section. The lens and cornea work together as a kind of "lens system".

The eyeball is only about 2.5 centimetres (1 inch) in diameter, and if focusing is to be precise this lens system must be free from flaws and very accurately positioned. Should the retina be only fractionally too far away, the focal point of rays from distant objects will fall short, so giving a blurred image. Conversely, if the retina is too close to the lens system (that is, if the eyeball is too short from front to rear), then the focal point of rays from nearby objects will fall, in theory at least, behind the retina, again producing a blurred image.

The refractive errors resulting from these two conditions are called **myopia** (short-sightedness) and **hypermetropia** (long-sightedness) respectively.

A third type of error, **astigmatism,** arises when there is a flaw in the shape of the cornea or, more rarely, in the shape of the lens. Unless the cornea is perfectly symmetrical, it will be unequally refractive and rays in differing planes will be brought to differing focal points, producing an image that will be only partly in focus, if at all (Figure 9).

Myopia, hypermetropia, and astigmatism can thus all be classed as refractive errors caused by malformation of the eyeball. The fourth common kind of refractive error, **presbyopia** (also called "old-age" sight and, confusingly, "far-sightedness"), is brought about because over the years the lens slowly loses its elasticity and hence its power to change shape during accommodation. In most people this process begins quite early in adulthood and is completed by the age of about 55 or 60, by which time all flexibility in the lens is lost.

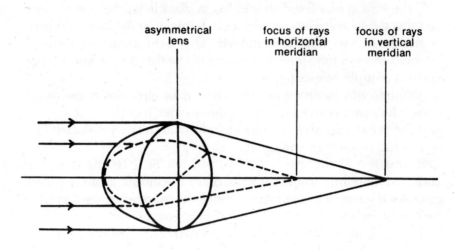

Figure 9: The principle of astigmatism

It is unusual for only one of the four common types of refractive error to be present in any given case. Most myopes, for example, have some degree of astigmatism also, and as a myope or a hypermetrope ages his condition is likely to be complicated by advancing presbyopia.

Floaters

These are the dark spots, tadpoles, and so on, which trouble many myopic and middle-aged people. They tend to come and go, and are most noticeable when reading or when the eyes are directed at some other bright surface, such as a blank white wall or the sky. In some cases the floaters appear to be stationary; in others they move with the tracking and searching movements of the eye, yet retain a certain momentum of their own when these movements cease.

Floaters are attributed to a fault in the vitreous humour. The vitreous humour is the fluid filling the vitreous body, and is similar to the aqueous humour, except that it has in addition a component of very fine fibrils. The fibrils give the vitreous humour a jelly-like consistency. In good health the jelly is firm, but in myopia or in later life it becomes more fluid. When this happens the fibrils can coagulate to some extent, and the shadows cast by the coagulations are perceived as floaters.

There may be other imperfections in the vitreous humour, not due to a deterioration of the jelly, which will also produce floaters, but these, while permanent, are usually transparent or nearly so and are much less annoying than the other kind.

Impaired coordination of the visual axes

In defective vision, no matter how minor the defect, there is almost always a deterioration in the action of the extrinsic muscles. One consequence of this is a loss of accuracy in coordinating the visual axes.

This accuracy is essential to good eyesight. If one eye. is functioning badly, or is focused on the wrong point, the brain suppresses its signals in favour of those from the other, taking the best information it can in order to build up the image. On the other hand, if both eyes are correctly brought to bear on the same point, they complement one another and the information reaching the brain is correspondingly more detailed and reliable.

The differences between the two sets of signals, left and right, form the basis of depth perception. The eyes are not spaced very far apart and, even if the vision is excellent, true stereoscopic perception rarely extends beyond about 45 metres (50 yards). Beyond that distance the signals from either eye are too similar to yield any information about depth. When true stereoscopic perception is impossible, we compensate to some extent with a pseudo-perception of depth based on our past knowledge of scale and perspective. It will be seen that, the more precise the control of the visual axes, the greater will be the range of true stereoscopic perception — with all the marvellous vividness and interest it brings to the visual field. When the use of the extrinsic muscles is poor, true depth perception many extend for only a few metres or less, or may even be completely absent.

Control of the visual axes is also important during accommodation. The angle between the visual axes gives a measure of the distance from the eyes to the object being perceived, and this is one source of the information that lets the eyes know where to refocus. This is not the only source, for a one-eyed man can also accommodate, but to be without it is to prevent the eyes from refocusing as swiftly as they should. And, conversely, changes in the focus of the eyes inform the extrinsic muscle system as to whether a change of angle is required. Thus faulty accommodation contributes to faulty use of the extrinsic muscles and vice versa.

Loss of foveal function

Faulty use of the extrinsic muscle impairs other functions too. The searching movements are coarsened so that objects in the visual field take longer to find, and tracking is slowed down so that fast-moving objects may be impossible to follow. Most serious of all, however, is impairment of the scanning action.

It is difficult to persuade someone with defective eyesight how much he is missing in life. The potential of the human visual system to convey detail is little short of astounding, and the quality of really good eyesight can only be described as breathtaking. Such quality is usually taken for granted by those people (mainly children) who possess it, and its loss takes place so insidiously that, except in the crudest way (through an awareness of decreasing focusing ability), it is hardly even noticed. When, with glasses, focusing ability is artificially restored, the wearer is sadly mistaken if he thinks he is seeing well again. With his new glasses he might be able to read the optician's chart, but there is very much more to good eyesight than that.

In one way, the eye works rather like a television camera. Instead of passively accepting the image cast by the lens upon the "film", as in an ordinary camera, there is an active scanning process in which the image is being continuously resolved into a multitude of tiny fragments before being reassembled in the brain. We see precisely only with the fovea, and we see most precisely of all with the foveola. The foveola is the point on the retina which must be scanned back and forth in order to resolve the greatest possible detail in the image.

An understanding of one of the principles involved can be gained from a study of photographs printed in newspapers, books, and magazines. If examined closely, it will be seen that the finished picture consists of a pattern of small dots. The smaller the size of the dots, the better the quality of reproduction. The smaller the functional area of the foveola (within the limits of the functioning of the retina), and the more accurately it can be scanned, the higher will be its power of resolution. The work of scanning is performed by the extrinsic muscles and the scanning action, as already noted, may be detected as a slight and continuous high-frequency tremor of the eyeball.

When the action of the extrinsic muscles deteriorates, the tremor becomes more clumsy. In effect, the "dots" get larger. The differentiation in function between foveola and fovea becomes less marked or is lost altogether. In more severe cases, there may be a loss of functional differentiation between the fovea and surrounding areas of the macula.

Photophobia

One of the effects of civilisation has been a reduction in the number of hours which most people spend out of doors. A worker in a shop, office, or factory may spend only a small proportion of his time exposed to the full spectrum and range of intensities of natural daylight. To this must be added the widespread effects of the idea that dark glasses are chic and confer on their owners a degree of sophistication that used to be the property of cigarette smokers. The same notion unfortunately prompts many people to have their prescription lenses unnecessarily tinted.

On leaving a brightly lit place (say when coming indoors on a sunny day), a phenomenon known as **dark adaptation** takes place in which there is an increase in the number of functioning rods and a decrease in the number of functioning cones. Although much of this change takes place quite rapidly, the full adaptation can take up to an hour. On leaving a dark place and coming into the light, the process is of course reversed.

The person who needlessly wears sunglasses will habitually be using too few cones in his retina. In time he becomes so adapted to dim light that exposure to the sun results in discomfort or even pain. The effect this has on accurate vision will be appreciated when it is remembered that the fovea contains only cones.

This type of photophobia is brought about simply by bad use. In the study of physiology there is an axiom which states: "Use makes the organ", or, more succinctly put, "Use it or lose it". Later we will see that this applies not only to light/dark adaptation, but also to the other functions of the eye — including accommodation.

"Noise" in the visual cortex

The last of the common defects we shall consider is to be found not in the eye, but in the brain.

When you cut off the supply of light to your visual system — when you shut your eyes and cover them with your hands — you should, once any after-images have faded, see nothing but blackness, absolute and infinitely deep. The chances are, though, that you see something else instead: perhaps a particulate swirling in grey or some other shade, or perhaps more elaborate, even kaleidoscopic, patterns. Sometimes these visions are so vivid that it is impossible to believe they are not somehow projected onto the eyelids; but, since no light is entering the eyes, the visions must be generated within the system. It is thought that they are a kind of interference in the visual cortex, background "noise" like the hissing of an amplifier. When you open your eyes again the interference does not go away: on it is superimposed the image of whatever you are seeing. It follows that, the worse the interference generated in the cortex, the more degraded will be the quality of the perceived image.

Bates placed great emphasis on the ability to "see black" and equated it with faultless eyesight. When black of equal depth is perceived at a distance and near to, and when the same quality of blackness can be held without effort in the memory, then, according to Dr Bates, the rest of the visual system is in perfect working order.

Refractive
Error

In order to understand any ailment, we must know whether it is congenital or acquired. Congenital defects are usually incurable, unless by surgery or other artificial means. By definition, they are determined by heredity — by the genetic inheritance of the individual concerned.

Acquired defects arise in various ways. There are those caused by such outside agencies as accident, infection, and contagion, and there are those (like ordinary obesity, drug addiction, most sorts of dental decay, much heart-disease, postural trouble, and so on) which are the result of bad use. That is, the individual, through various bad habits, practised consciously or otherwise, brings the affliction on himself. In these cases, if the manner of use can be improved, then, providing things have not gone too far, the natural restorative and recuperative powers of the body are likely, given time, to effect a complete or partial cure.

Actually it is not as straightforward as that. Genes can strongly influence one's predisposition to acquired defects — even to those caused by outside agencies. Strictly speaking, perhaps, most defects can be said to have some sort of genetic involvement, and it might be better to reclassify as acquired defects those over which the individual has, potentially at least, a measure of control. None the less, the distinction between "congenital" and "acquired" defects is a real one, and for simplicity's sake we will allow it to stand.

Is refractive error congenital or acquired? According to the medical profession, it can be both, but the primary causes are congenital. The medical profession would list the causes of refractive error as follows:

1 malformation of the eyeball (congenital);
2 hardening of the lens with age (congenital);
3 incipient cataract and other pathological conditions (congenital or acquired); and
4 changes in the refractive properties of the aqueous or vitreous (congenital or acquired).

Objections to the orthodox view

Let us for the moment presume to question the accepted view. Is it possible that our doctors are, at least in part, mistaken about the causes of refractive error? Is it possible that the theories on which much of modern ophthalmology is based are unsound and lacking the authority of a truly scientific approach?

The scientific tradition since the Renaissance has been based on a single method: that of hypothesis and experiment. A hypothesis is formed in order to explain a number of observations. The next step, of course, is to test the hypothesis with experiments which systematically gather further observations. These further observations may confirm the hypothesis, in which case it can be restated as a fact. On the other hand, if the experimenter finds just one observation which does not fit the hypothesis, then the whole thing must be reconsidered, modified, or even abandoned altogether.

Are there any observations which do not fit the present theories accounting for refractive error?

Consider myopia, which is attributed, in the overwhelming majority of cases, to an eye that is too large. We should expect to find that this error, arising from a congenital physical defect, is pretty well constant from day to day and week to week and, in young adults at least, from month to month and year to year. We should also expect that myopic children would become more short-sighted as their eyes, and the rest of their bodies, grew in size, and that this increase in myopia would come to a decisive halt on maturity. Yet this is not the experience of very many adult myopes, who find their prescriptions changing at various times and at irregular intervals long after developmental growth has ceased.

In the absence of any eye disease which would allow an explanation under heading 3 above, which of the other causes might we invoke to explain changes in myopia in adults? The size of the eyeball is held to be invariable, so 1 is obviously not it. Could the lens be hardening with age? But that would tend to make the eye more far-sighted, not more myopic, and the usual course of events is for adult myopia to get worse. Since we have already ruled out 3, the answer must be 4: the refractive properties of the aqueous or vitreous must be changing. But this is so rare a condition that it would be absurd to ascribe so many cases of progressive myopia in adults to this cause.

Consider also the common experience of myopes — indeed of anybody — when fitted with a new pair of glasses. They are warned that they must expect to have to get used to the new lenses, that there will be an initial period of discomfort or unpleasantness. Why? If, as we are assured, the presence or absence of a corrective lens has no effect on the eye (beyond temporarily allowing it to focus properly), if the eye can be treated as an inert optical device with invariable refractive properties, why should it be necessary to have to adjust to new glasses? The feeling of discomfort often takes the form of a sort of muscular strain, the sensation that one's eyes are almost being "pulled out on their stalks". What is this sensation, and what causes it?

It is also a common experience among myopes that glasses tend to make the eyesight worse. To take a specific example, an acquaintance of mine was given, late in his childhood, a pair of National Health Service glasses to correct mild myopia. The frames formerly supplied by the British welfare state were extremely basic and many people considered them unattractive. In consequence he wore his glasses only intermittently and his eyesight remained stable for a number of years. Then, in his late twenties, when he became more prosperous, he decided to order a private pair with similar lenses but lighter frames. Having spent a good deal of money on his new glasses, he began to wear them regularly. He soon found that his eyesight was worse and that he was now dependent on his glasses. This deterioration in his sight took place long after he had stopped growing; and it is interesting to note that it coincided exactly with the acquisition of his new glasses. Similar cases, whether among myopes, hypermetropes, or presbyopes, are by no means unusual. How can they be explained?

How also does one explain the fact that people with severe myopia (whose eyes are supposed to be overlarge) develop a curious and characteristic "mole-eyed" appearance? Their eyes look small and weak when they take off their glasses, which, naturally, they always seem eager to put on again. Yet, should their glasses be lost or broken, this mole-eyed appearance gradually begins, after a few days, to diminish. Quite often, too, the vision begins to improve, if only marginally. If myopia is congenital, and the wearing of glasses makes no difference to the eyes, it is impossible to account for these observations and we are driven to the conclusion that the present hypotheses must be lacking.

Although we have considered in detail the case of myopia, objections may also be raised to the orthodox explanations of the other kinds of refractive error. The medical profession freely allows that astigmatism can change with time, which is difficult to understand if we are to accept that astigmatism is caused by congenital malformation of the cornea (or, rarely, the lens). Hypermetropia, like myopia, can also change after adulthood has been attained; the difference here, however, is that younger eyes are said to be able to compensate for hypermetropia by use of the ciliary muscle. As the lens hardens, this compensation is said to become progressively less effective. Thus it is less easy to argue convincingly against the orthodox theory of hypermetropia. The same is true of presbyopia. Without statistical evidence, it is not valid to advance as an argument the subjective observation that presbyopia tends to develop earlier in underactive individuals, or that, in less frantic cultures than our own, old people often seem to live out their days without ever needing glasses, even though they still engage in close work of various kinds.

Thus the most convincing arguments are those that can be advanced against the orthodox accounts of myopia and astigmatism. If these objections hold firm, we are then entitled to question the rest of orthodox theory as it applies to the other refractive errors too.

Most of the objections to the orthodox explanation of myopia can be understood only if we reject the idea that glasses have no lasting effect on the eyes. This strongly suggests that vision can change through causes not currently recognised by the medical profession. What might those causes be?

The Bates hypothesis

Bates postulated that the fundamental cause of refractive error is what he called "strain". He believed that strain interferes with the unconscious habits of good vision. Refractive error, according to the Bates hypothesis, far from being congenital and incurable, is an acquired defect. Provided the bad habits can be replaced with good, and provided the right conditions can be created in which recovery can take place, there is every chance that refractive error can be alleviated.

From his writings it emerges that this "strain" is of two sorts: emotional disturbance, and the self-induced strain caused by *trying* to see (instead of letting the visual process operate in a relaxed and unimpeded way).

We will look first at emotional disturbance. By this is meant the instability brought on by such negative feelings as boredom, worry, fear, grief, and so on. The effects of these feelings, and the capacity to experience them, will vary greatly with the personality of the individual concerned, and so we would expect wide variation in the response of different people to the same conditions.

In Chapter 2 we saw that vision is a function of the cerebral cortex, and is a creative process closely allied to imagination and memory. In light of this, it is not unreasonable to suggest that a disturbance elsewhere in the cortex, in the areas concerned with thought and feelings, might have an influence on the visual process. It is certainly true to say that emotional disturbance can upset other functions of the cortex. A child in school, for example, is unlikely to be at its most receptive in a state of boredom or unhappiness. The creative processes of memory and imagination (seen at their best, perhaps, in the composition of a work of art or literature) appear to function most efficiently in a mind that is calm and unharassed.

The first part of the Bates hypothesis, then, states that — in some manner which ultimately interferes with the mechanism of accommodation — emotional disturbance adversely affects the visual process. If this is true, the hypothesis may be enlarged at this stage to include certain predictions.

If emotional disturbance makes refractive error worse, then presumably a return to emotional stability will make it better again.

But what happens if this process is interrupted—what happens if, in response to a deterioration in eyesight, glasses are acquired and used? We know that accommodation is automatically and involuntarily controlled by feedback from the brain. If the perceived image is in focus, then the brain is satisfied that the mechanism of accommodation is working properly. Hence glasses will effectively short-circuit the feedback process and, once the negative conditions that gave rise to the emotional disturbance have passed, the return to better eyesight will be arrested. For, in order to see clearly through a lens, the eye must continuously produce the very refractive error the lens is designed to overcome. Thus we would expect refractive error to be confirmed and perpetuated by wearing glasses, and we would expect that only when the glasses are left off will the vision have a chance to recover.

Under this hypothesis, refractive error is not only taken to be a *symptom* of emotional disturbance; it can also be a *source* of emotional disturbance, of anxiety and stress. As a broad generality, the myope tends to be bookish, introspective, and shy, to retreat into the safety of the world on which he can focus; while the hypermetrope's life is unbalanced in the opposite way. And of course, the physical handicap of bad eyesight is itself a source of stress.

In addition, we must not forget what happens during a visit to the optician's. There, surrounded by unfamiliar and rather intimidating-looking equipment, the patient is placed in an adjustable chair, the lights are dimmed, and the optician, after examining the eyes with his instruments, asks the patient to read the test chart and answer questions. The patient, misguidedly believing that his replies will determine his prescription, is afraid that a "wrong" answer will ultimately be bad for his eyes. The examination is therefore made in circumstances in which the patient's eyesight is likely to be temporarily, if only slightly, worse than usual. The result is that he is prescribed lenses which are slightly stronger than he actually needs: his eyes must learn to get used to them, and his vision deteriorates accordingly.

So far the Bates hypothesis accords well with the observations made earlier about one type of refractive error and the effect that glasses have on it. What of the second component of the strain that Dr Bates cites as a source of refractive error—what of the strain induced by trying to see?

In the performance of its various functions, the human frame (in its ideal state) works best without conscious intervention. The act of walking, for instance, should be performed automatically. As soon as the mind tries to think about the mechanics of walking, as soon as it tries to decide what goes where and which action follows which, as soon, in short, as one *tries* to walk, then the whole performance goes wrong. The same is true of the act of seeing. If the mind tries to interfere with those aspects of seeing which ought, so to speak, to be left in the care of the autopilot, the result is always bad.

By the very structure of the extrinsic muscles, the eyes are inherently prone to this kind of interference. The extrinsic muscles contain both striped and smooth tissue and are subject to conscious as well as involuntary control. This is especially unfortunate for the scanning action which, crucial to eyesight, is the only exclusively automatic function of the extrinsic muscles. The other types of eye movement—control of the visual axes, tracking, and searching—all respond in some measure to the will.

Accommodation can also be consciously influenced. For a few moments at a time it is possible to exaggerate whatever refractive error one habitually possesses—to make oneself more short-sighted or long-sighted or astigmatic, as the case may be. And of course the eyelids, which normally blink quite automatically, are subject to immediate conscious control.

Whenever we wish to use any of our senses especially acutely, we suppress as distracting all unnecessary movements of the body. Someone trying to hear a faint sound is apt to hold himself perfectly still, then turn his head in such a way that one ear is held in the most advantageous position; he is likely to look downwards, towards the ground, in order to suppress any incoming visual signals, and concentrate all his attention on his hearing. For a while he is almost like a statue. Even his breathing becomes shallower; it may even, temporarily, be suspended altogether.

A similar sort of thing happens when one tries to make out some faint or unfamiliar sight. The breathing and other bodily movements are suppressed, the rate of blinking decreases, and the eyes are fixed in a stare. Should this staring become a regular habit, the danger is that persistent fixing of the extrinsic muscles will upset the delicate mechanism of the scanning action. Loss of mobility in tracking and searching will spill over into loss of mobility in scanning and, since the tone of adjacent muscle systems is related, into loss of mobility in the mechanism of accommodation also.

Unfortunately for us, the civilised way of life makes it very tempting to acquire such habits. When we look at something and give it our attention, that attention may be given in one of two ways. In *The Art of Seeing,* Aldous Huxley makes the distinction between "spontaneous" and "voluntary" attention. The former is the unforced attention that any animal (including the human one) gives to whatever catches its eye; the latter is the kind that is given under conscious control. To quote Huxley: "A small boy studying algebra exhibits voluntary attention — that is, if he exhibits any attention at all. The same boy playing a game exhibits spontaneous attention. Voluntary attention is always associated with effort, and tends more or less rapidly to produce fatigue."

Successful seeing depends on free mobility of the attention as well as of the eyes. By forcing ourselves, for some ulterior purpose, to attend to things in which we are not really interested, we are interfering with the natural process of perception. For the human species, this misuse is an unavoidable consequence of our faculty of foresight. It is hazardous for the eyes rather than harmful. Harm only accrues when the misuse becomes habitual and persists into those circumstances where the attention given should be of the spontaneous variety.

Trying also degrades eyesight in another way. We have already established that seeing is an essentially creative process akin to imagination and memory, and any creative process is impaired by trying. If one tries to remember a name it usually proves elusive; only later, when the trying stops, does the name come effortlessly to mind. Creative work, whether it be cooking a soufflé or writing a symphony, is paradoxically at its best when the strain to succeed is absent. This is illustrated by a Japanese story* about the master calligrapher Kosen, who had been asked to prepare a draft of the words *The First Principle,* which were to be carved above the gateway at Obaku temple in Kyoto. The work was not going well, for in his studio Kosen had a pupil who was keenly critical of his master's efforts. Draft followed draft until Kosen had wasted 84 sheets of

*Paul Reps, *Zen Flesh, Zen Bones* (Penguin Books, 1971)

paper. Finally, when the pupil stepped outside for a moment, Kosen thought "Now's my chance" and then, with a mind free from distraction, wrote: *The First Principle.* "A masterpiece," the pupil declared, and the characters can be seen at the temple to this day.

An alternative method of accommodation?

To recapitulate, the Bates hypothesis states that the source of refractive error is strain, whether caused indirectly, by emotional disturbance, or directly, by trying to see. The hypothesis seems reasonable enough, at least superficially. It already has the edge on the orthodox hypotheses in that it is capable of explaining observations which otherwise would remain inexplicable. And doubtless, as it has been described so far, its ideas are broadly acceptable to the medical profession. The stumbling block comes only when we must propose a new theory of accommodation to replace or supplement the one that has been found lacking. This is where the Bates method and orthodoxy usually part company.

The power of the method to improve every type of refractive error, astigmatism and presbyopia included, strongly suggests that Bates was right in believing that the eye can alter its shape and thereby its refractive properties. If, however, we reject his idea that the extrinsic muscles accomplish this operation, what other possibilities remain?

The eye is like a sphere filled with fluid. In order for its shape to change, some kind of pressure must be exerted on the wall of the sphere, either by muscular action (as in Bates's original idea), or hydrostatically, by a change in the volume of the fluid.

Looking at a diagram of the eye (Figure 1), where might we find tissues capable of exerting such pressure? There is nothing in the sclera, choroid, or retina capable of independent movement; the only musculature found within the eyeball itself, besides that of the iris, is that of the ciliary body, and it is impossible to see how that might influence the shape of the eye in the necessary manner. We are left with the fluid, which consists of the three optical media: the lens, the aqueous, and the vitreous. The first two seem unlikely candidates. The Bates method can alleviate presbyopia (when the lens has lost all its elasticity), and the aqueous humour is a clear fluid without any structure whatever. The vitreous, on the other hand, although consisting of 98.5 per cent water, does have a more or less definite structure, for which no function has ever been proposed.

Besides water, the vitreous contains a protein of the collagen-gelatin type, and a polysaccharide (a sugar with a long, chain-like molecule), hyaluronic acid. The protein is present in the form of a dense network of fine fibrils.

Microscope preparations of the human vitreous are extremely difficult to make. They do not take stains well and are liable to artefacts — optical illusions produced by the method of preparation. Nonetheless there is a constancy of appearance which suggests that there is a real internal structure. It is believed that the fibrils cross each other without forming actual connections. At more or less regular intervals, spherical thickenings occur on the fibrils. These are believed to be caused by the fibril itself thickening at that point. The vitreous lies in contact with the retina but generally is not firmly adherent to it. There is firm attachment at the optic disc and at the **ora serrata,** the rim of the retina. In youth especially, it also adheres to the lens and to the macula. The attachment at the ora serrata is especially strong and the origin of all the vitreous fibrils can be traced to this region.

The role of the vitreous fibrils is open to speculation. It has always been assumed that their function is one of support, but, since the eye maintains its shape by hydrostatic pressure, the fluid in the vitreous would alone, presumably, provide all the support necessary.

Might the vitreous be involved in accommodation? Its contents occupy the greater part of the eye: if the vitreous could change its shape or volume, the change would be transmitted directly to the surrounding portion of the sclera and hydrostatically, through the aqueous, to the cornea.

The microscopic appearance of the fibrils seems to suggest that the network might be able to alter its shape by contraction and subsequent relaxation of individual fibrils. Since the vitreous is firmly attached at the ora serrata and at the optic disc, contraction and relaxation of the fibrils would allow the eye, under hydrostatic pressure, to modify its shape. If one part of the network habitually contracted more than another, this differential contraction would give rise to an irregularity in the cornea — to astigmatism. Control of the contractions would come presumably from the retina, or perhaps from the optic disc. It is hard to see, though, how a structure as tenuous as the vitreous network could have the necessary mechanical strength. There might instead be some chemical change going on which would alter the permeability of the network and hence the volume of the vitreous as a whole. A reduction in volume would have the same effect as a contraction of the fibrils — the eye would shorten from front to back. The idea of chemical change, however, seems unlikely when the rapidity of accommodation is taken into account.

Whatever the truth of the matter, and whether or not the vitreous is a factor in accommodation, experience of the Bates method has convinced me that the eye can indeed change its shape. In the early stages of my Bates training I became aware, during flashes of near-perfect vision, of a slight pulling sensation inside the eye. The pulling seemed to be located in the region of the eye occupied by the ciliary body, or by the ora serrata — I cannot say which. The sensation and the clear vision lasted only until I blinked, when both disappeared. I no longer have the pulling sensation, but the precise quality of my vision still varies, as it were, from blink to blink. The eyelids, being brought across the cornea, must modify the shape of the eyeball.

Myopes have a habit of squinting when they wish to see better. It has been suggested that the improvement comes because, by a reduction in aperture, the eye is turned into a sort of pin-hole camera. This cannot be the full answer, because even a slight squint, leaving the whole of the pupil visible, can bring an improvement. It is much more likely that the pressure of the eyelids squeezes the eyeball so that it becomes marginally shorter from front to back. Thus the eyelids can modify a shape which has just been set by the primary focusing device — whether it is the vitreous, Bates's extrinsic muscles, or something else entirely. The lens is probably a secondary device, rather like the fine focus on a microscope — useful for bringing extra precision to the image, but by no means essential.

In my own mind I am satisfied that the present theory of accommodation is inadequate and sooner or later will have to be revised. At this stage all that can be usefully said is that there is already a mass of evidence to suggest that an alternative mechanism is at work: the evidence of the many thousands of people who have improved their vision by means of the Bates method. For those who demand a theoretical explanation of every remedial treatment they undergo, this will not be enough, but for the ordinary person worried about his eyesight and without the leisure to wait until science comes up with another theory, it makes little difference *how* something works as long as it *does* work, and work — for the majority — the Bates method most certainly does.

PART TWO

Beginning
with the Method

In this part of the book the techniques of the Bates method will be described in detail. Each technique is aimed mainly at faults in one area of the visual system, but the techniques also reinforce and complement one another, so that in every case of defective vision it is advisable to explore them all. From what has been said earlier it will be seen that much of the method is entirely consistent with orthodox knowledge of the way that eyesight works; the rest is similarly consistent, but with the Bates hypothesis rather than the orthodox one.

It is recommended that you read straight through Part Two before trying out any of the techniques. Then, if you are persuaded that they make sense, reread each chapter in turn and experiment at your own pace. At the end of this, if you still feel there may be something in the Bates method for you, commit yourself to a period of not less than six weeks (two months would be better) in which you are prepared to give it a chance. During this time you are entitled to be as sceptical as you like, provided you do your best to keep an open mind. Once this period is up, if you feel you are getting nowhere you will at least have investigated the method to your satisfaction and can safely reject it.

On the other hand, if you experience an improvement in your vision, no matter how temporary or slight, you will have demonstrated that the orthodox explanation of your refractive error is unreliable. At this stage it is suggested that you commit yourself, with rather less scepticism, to a further period of six weeks or two months, during which you are likely to find yourself becoming convinced that the method works. If with this conviction you can make a firm decision to carry the method through, you will have at least a 75 per cent chance of meeting with partial or complete success. By partial success I mean a reduced dependence on glasses and a weaker prescription than the one you have at the moment.

The obvious first step towards rehabilitating the eyes is to discard one's glasses. It should be emphasised here that the ophthalmic profession is agreed that you do no harm whatever if you choose not to wear glasses that have been prescribed for refractive error.

If you can dispense with your glasses from the start, so much the better. The more you wear them, the slower your progress will be. Bates was quite insistent that glasses should never be worn by anyone hoping for success with his method, but this is something of a counsel of perfection. If the eyesight is very weak, a sudden "cold turkey" might produce strain, and strain is the very thing the method sets out to avoid. Moreover, glasses are often essential to carrying out one's job of work, and, in cases of even fairly mild myopia, to drive without glasses would be not only illegal but insane.

As far as refractive error is concerned, the effect of contact lenses on the eyes is much the same as that of glasses. Because contact lenses are not usually so quick to apply and remove as glasses, they are apt to be worn more continuously and to that extent are more harmful. It might be worth considering going over to a pair of glasses for a while, if you have them.

To begin with, you should aim to remove your glasses at any time you do not actually need them. The worse your eyesight and the longer you have been wearing glasses, the harder this will be. If your eyesight is so poor that you feel helpless without them, work out a timetable according to which, each day, you wear your glasses for 15 or 20 minutes less, and at the end of each week make a note of how many hours in all your glasses have been worn.

The act of putting on one's glasses in the morning can easily become automatic. Not to do it will feel odd at first. And then, especially in social situations, a lack of glasses can give an unpleasant feeling of vulnerability. Overcoming this feeling, if you experience it, is all part of the process, and when you have achieved it you will know that you have already made an important step forward.

Then there will be questions from people who are not accustomed to seeing you without your glasses. Family and close friends might be sympathetic; others may well scoff. In the early weeks and months you will be sceptical enough on your own account without having to convince anyone else. I suggest that you be very selective about whom you discuss the method with. Your investigation of it is a personal matter; questions about the absence of your glasses should be answered as economically as possible. Nobody will very much care, and later, if and when you find that the method works, you can afford to be more open and confident. Incidentally, however sure you may be of the value of the method, never try to convert anyone to it. Mention it in conversation by all means, but at the first sign of indifference or hostility let the subject drop. The emotional problems that cause some people to wear glasses in the first place may not allow them to listen impartially to your advice, however well-intentioned it may be.

At this point you might begin to ask yourself some questions about your own emotional life, especially in the past. Remember if you can when your first and succeeding pairs of glasses were prescribed. Were the preceding months relaxed and happy, or was there perhaps some event or series of events which might have been upsetting? If you were first given glasses as a schoolchild, were you completely happy at school, or might there have been one or more teachers whom you particularly feared or disliked? Did you find your schooldays restrictive and boring; was there too much emphasis on competition and exams?

Any thoughts you may have about these and similar questions should be jotted down on paper, as should any notes you want to make about your experience with the method. It is a useful plan to keep a special diary for this purpose — an exercise book will do — so that in your more doubting moments you have documentary evidence to rely on. In this diary you can also record details of your practice sessions and standards of visual acuity attained.

T W O

Palming

The central tenet of the Bates hypothesis is that refractive error is caused by strain: the logical antidote is to rest the eyes by closing them for a while. This is something that everyone does when tired or when trying to get over an unpleasant experience. If the experience is sufficiently disturbing, the natural tendency is to cover the eyes with the hands as well.

Studies of the electrical discharges of the cerebral cortex go some way towards explaining this. The electrical discharges take the form of rhythmic patterns, or brain waves, which are of several kinds. Beta waves are generated when the visual field is patterned (that is, when the eyes are open in the normal way), but when the visual field is uniform (when the eyes are closed) the brain waves change to the calmer alpha type.

The simple idea of resting the eyes by closing them is basic to the Bates method. Dr Bates coined for it the term "palming". The eyes are gently closed and covered with the palms in such a way that all light is excluded and no pressure is applied to the eyeballs. The heels of the hands rest lightly on the cheekbones and the fingers on the forehead. Palming is usually done while seated. The elbows should be supported, either on a table in front of you or on a thick cushion or two in your lap.

While palming, you should feel entirely comfortable, safe and warm. Choose if you can a quiet time and a place where you are not likely to be disturbed. Become conscious of and do your best to relax any undue tension in the muscles of your face, neck, shoulders, and the rest of your body. Listen to the radio if you wish, or just allow the mind to wander, keeping it away from anything unpleasant. If stressful thoughts intrude, push them aside to be dealt with later.

Remain with the eyes shut for several minutes. The exact period that suits you best has to be found by trial and error; five minutes is about right, and four should be regarded as a minimum. It can be difficult to judge the passage of time, and some such device as a non-ticking cook's timer, or one of those electronic watches or pocket calculators which incorporate an alarm, is very useful.

Palming like this should be repeated from three to five times in succession and forms the basis of your daily practice period. Once or twice in the period you might like, rather than merely allowing the mind to wander, to try some visualisation. This is a powerful technique which relies on the fact that all mental activity is accompanied by corresponding physical rehearsal. Thus if you imagine that you are speaking, or even if you frame your thoughts in terms of words rather than abstractions, there are minute but measurable movements of the vocal apparatus; if you imagine you are clenching and unclenching your fist, all the muscles involved undergo fractional changes of tension. When you see with your mind's eye, the real eyes respond in a similar way, except that, as the eyes are even more intimately related to the mind than, say, the muscles of the arm, the changes are likely to be more pronounced. The advantage of mental seeing is that the mind's eye has no refractive error and forms a model for the real eyes to emulate.

Visualisation is also valuable exercise for the memory and imagination. With your mind's eye examine some outdoor scene, remembered, imagined, or a mixture of both, that gives you particular pleasure. Allow your gaze to take in details both in the distance and near to, changing the focus swiftly and easily as various objects attract your interest. If you are short-sighted, pay special attention to distant scenes, and if you are long-sighted or presbyopic, pay special attention to objects close at hand.

It might be wondered why an ordinary night's sleep does not have the same effect as palming and visualisation. The eyes are closed, and during dreams there is plenty of imagery to work on. If the sleep is sound, the eyes are indeed rested and the eyesight often tends to be better on rising, but for many people sleep produces a degree of eyestrain. While dreaming the eyes perform rapid and random movements, there is no control of the memory or imagination, and very often the dreams themselves are in some measure disturbing. In all, dreaming would seem to be associated with a turmoil in the cortex which is the opposite of the calm, easy state in which the eyes work best. If you suffer from eyestrain during sleep, the Bates technique of "long swinging" (see p. 63), practised just before retiring, may be of value.

Palming can and should also be practised for shorter periods at any odd moment. Even a few seconds of palming will help to keep the eyes refreshed and the mind relaxed. In circumstances where palming with both hands would be embarrassing, palm each eye individually, or, if you feel that even this would draw unwelcome attention to yourself, merely shut the eyes as if dozing. When watching television, make use of commercial breaks for palming.

The quality of the blackness that you see when palming is a measure of the state of your vision. Although in his book Dr Bates suggests that the imagination should be actively used to intensify the blackness perceived, this is a practice which can give rise to strain, and so was not advocated by other teachers, or indeed by Bates himself in the latter part of his life. It was found that it was better to let uniformity and blackness of the visual field develop of themselves as a response to general improvement of the eyesight. Nonetheless, it is worth experimenting briefly with "seeing black" while palming, for in a few cases this technique can be very effective indeed. Take as the subject of your visualisation the blackest things you can think of — black fur, black velvet, Indian ink, and so on — and picture them in rapid succession. Or rapidly progress through the letters of the alphabet, imagining each one as being very black and distinct before moving on to the next. When you reach Z, compare the blackness of the letter with the blackness of your visual field. If the letter is blacker, let it merge with the background and the whole should become blacker. This process can be repeated again and again to produce a yet deeper black.

A variant of it engages the eyesight as well as the imagination, and strengthens the use of the memory. Study one of the letters from the large test chart (Chart A), at whatever distance you see it best. For some reason an angular letter such as an F or H seems most effective for this. Memorise every detail of its form: the width of the limbs, their relationship with one another, the shape and pattern of the background of white. Above all remember how black the letter is. Then cover the eyes and see how much of your memory you can retain. Do not struggle at this; do not try to concentrate. If the letter disappears at once, so be it. But, if you find it remains, go on to the next stage, which is to imagine the letter imprinted in the deepest possible black on the far side of a matt white cylinder. Let the cylinder slowly rotate on its long axis until the letter comes into view. Then forget the cylinder. Allow it to vanish, leaving just the letter against the background of your visual field. If the letter is blacker than the field, let it merge as before.

All these techniques, and indeed all the techniques of the Bates method, are effective in some cases but not in others. It is up to you to find out which ones suit you and which do not. A few people even have difficulty with simple palming and must achieve a degree of improvement with the other techniques before returning to it. At the start of your Bates training, give each technique a trial. If you find it unhelpful, go on to another, bearing in mind always that later on you might like to come back to it and try again.

C · H · A · P · T · E · R

THREE

Sunning

The evolution of the human species has been going on for millions of years. For all but a tiny fraction of that time, man was a hunter and gatherer, living in intimate relationship with the landscape. Even after the coming of agriculture, indeed until the early years of this century, most human beings began their day at dawn and ended it at dusk or soon afterwards. Man is essentially a diurnal creature, and his cone-rich retina works best in sunlight. Deprived of sun, the retina eventually adapts and becomes pathologically hypersensitive to even quite ordinary light intensities.

This oversensitivity to light, or photophobia, is both a defect in itself and a sign of disorder elsewhere in the visual system. It can range from the mildest sort, such that there is a tendency to squint when facing the sun, to a serious condition in which the eyes must be permanently protected with dark glasses. In nearly every case photophobia is acquired rather than congenital, and originates in the fact that the majority of us now spend much of our lives indoors. If photophobia can be overcome the eye is relieved of a great deal of strain, and this in turn encourages normal functioning generally.

The Bates technique for alleviating photophobia is called sunning, and consists simply of taking sunshine on the closed lids. In this way the retina is accustomed to progressively brighter light, until the stage is reached where the eye can function efficiently over the entire range of normally encountered light intensities. The warmth of the sun and the therapeutic properties of its rays also have a profound and beneficial effect on the health of the eyes and on the ability to relax them.

49

Begin if you can by taking half a minute of sun, palm until the after-images have substantially faded, and repeat two or three times. At the next sunning session increase the period slightly and repeat it an extra time, building up over the weeks and months to a maximum of 20 minutes of sun in all.

If you are so photophobic that you find it uncomfortable to let the sun shine on your closed lids, face the brightest part of the sky that you can. At the next session approach the sun a little more, until for a brief spell you can take the sun without discomfort on the lids. If even the brightness of the sky is too much, begin with artificial light, bringing the lamp gradually closer until you feel ready to start sunning outdoors.

Sunning sessions can be held two or three times a day if desired. When there is no sun, use artificial light instead. The lamp bulb should be of the ordinary household type (150 watts), or, for preference, a 100 watt silver-backed reflector spotlight (cheaply obtainable from any lighting store). Such a spotlight is useful for other Bates work too, so it might be worth getting one if you do not already have something suitable. Do not use fluorescent light for sunning, and under no circumstances use an infrared or ultraviolet lamp.

Sit with the lamp at eye level and at a comfortable distance, bringing it a few inches closer at each succeeding session until its brightness on the closed lids approximates to that of the sun. If you prefer, position the lamp behind your shoulder, angled so that you can reflect the light into your face with a mirror held in your lap. This arrangement is not to be recommended for outdoor sunning, because reflected sunlight has slightly different properties from the real thing.

Whether you are sunning indoors or out, keep your head slowly moving so that the light is distributed evenly across each retina. The simplest way to do this is to swing the head from side to side through 90 degrees or a little more, taking about 7–10 seconds to move from one side to the other. Vary the movement if you like by swinging the head so that, if a paintbrush were attached to your nose, you would be painting a circle, an infinity sign, a figure-of-eight, or any other geometrical figure that pleases you. Every few swings, reverse the direction of travel. During sunning you should feel yourself becoming agreeably drowsy, infused by the warm glow coming through your eyelids. Let the glow spread until it seems to take over your whole body. If, however, you ever find sunning uncomfortable or unpleasant, stop immediately.

Some accounts of the Bates method mention a more advanced technique in which the sun is taken directly on the retina. This open-eyed sunning sounds more alarming than it really is. No one in his right mind would dream of staring at the sun, for this would cause severe damage to the eyes, and perhaps even blindness. Brief and extremely cautious exposure of the retina to the sun's disc, however, is quite safe. One eye is sunned at a time, the other being covered with the hand. Turn the head quickly so that the sun sweeps across the retina (the turn of the head takes only a couple of seconds), blinking rapidly and easily as you do so. Repeat with the other eye, and then palm until all after-images have faded.

Open-eyed sunning is undoubtedly of value for some people in the later stages of their Bates training, as it removes the final traces of photophobia, but in the ordinary way its benefits are not noticeably greater than those of closed-eyed sunning, and it can cause strain. It is probably best left alone, at least to begin with. In any event it should only be used sparingly and responsibly. The technique is described here mainly for the sake of completeness.

Like palming, sunning can also be done at odd moments, whenever the opportunity presents itself and you have a few seconds to spare.

It goes without saying that, whenever possible, sunglasses are to be avoided. After Bates training you are less likely to feel the need of them anyway, but if ever you do, a wide-brimmed hat or sunshade will probably give all the protection necessary. In temperate latitudes, sunglasses are usually only needed in conditions of exceptional glare (during prolonged exposure to sunlit snow, for example); in the tropics, however, and particularly for Caucasians and others whose forebears evolved in more temperate zones, sunglasses may be required more often. In these circumstances lenses of the best quality should be used. Cheap sunglasses, besides distorting the image, cannot be relied upon to give adequate protection from excessive ultraviolet radiation.

The squinting and grimacing that accompany photophobia can become a habit that persists even after the photophobia itself has gone. Whenever you catch yourself squinting, ask yourself whether you really need to do it; allow your face muscles to relax, and take pleasure in your new and easy relationship with the sun. Squinting is not only unattractive in itself, but it also aggravates the formation of wrinkles and makes you look older than you should.

Sunning is aimed specifically at daylight vision. It is worth giving a little thought to your night sight as well, especially if your work or hobby involves vision in dim light. Once in a while, delay switching on the lamps in the evening for half an hour or longer. Notice how, as darkness gathers and the rods take over from the cones, detail and colour and, to some extent, depth perception gradually vanish.

Do not try to make out detail, because this is futile and causes strain. In fact you have a better chance of resolving detail if you do as the astronomers do when they wish to pick out a very faint star. Rather than staring straight at it, they look off to one side, allowing its light to fall outside the macula and in a part of the retina where the rods outnumber cones.

C·H·A·P·T·E·R

FOUR

Fusion

We now come to the part of the Bates method aimed at improving the use of the extrinsic muscles. Tracking, searching, and scanning are helped by the techniques covered in the chapters on mobility; fusion techniques, given here, will improve control of the visual axes.

Together with the accommodation drills to be described later, fusion techniques come as close as anything else in the Bates method to what is normally understood by the term "eye exercises". In one sense they are indeed eye exercises, because the extrinsic muscles and the mechanism of accommodation are strengthened by them, but to say that they are nothing more is to simplify what they achieve. They make use of conscious control in order to improve control on the unconscious plane. This principle is basic to the whole of the Bates method, and runs through nearly every one of its techniques.

Fusion drills are very simple. The first may be used as a test to determine whether your fusion (control of the visual axes) is faulty and needs further work.

Pencil fusion

Take a pencil and hold it up straight in front of you and about 45 centimetres (18 inches) from your face. Look at the pencil, and then allow your eyes to refocus in the distance beyond it (on the far wall if you are indoors). You should now be able to see two blurred pencils, like gateposts one on either side of the point you are looking at. The two pencils should be equally plain. If they

53

are not, if you can only see one, or if the point in the distance also appears double, then your fusion is certainly faulty.

If you can only see one pencil, shut either eye alternately to find out which is the weaker. Now cover the stronger eye and look at the pencil again. Refocus in the distance and memorise where the pencil comes in relation to the distant view. Uncover the stronger eye. Does it dominate the weaker one completely; does the pencil immediately switch sides? Or are you able to retain the weaker eye's pencil, at least for a moment or two?

Similarly, practise covering the stronger eye if both pencils are visible but one is clearer than the other. If the distant point is also double, practise with one eye at a time, focusing first on the pencil and then in the distance, bringing your focus back to the pencil. Repeat this routine three times with each eye, then try both together. Don't worry if you have difficulty with this or with any of the fusion drills. They will all come eventually, aided by your progress with palming and sunning.

Once you are familiar with pencil fusion in this form, try two-pencil fusion. The following explanation sounds rather involved, but is easy to understand in practice. For two-pencil fusion you need some definite reference point in the distance: any object that will fit conveniently into the "gateway". Hold one pencil up at arm's length, and another a few inches from your face. Practise making two gateways, one enclosing the other and both enclosing the reference point. Aim to make each of the "four" pencils equally plain, although the nearer gateway will of course be more blurred. Now focus on the further pencil. You should find that your reference point has doubled: each of the two should appear equally plain. Bring your focus back to the nearer pencil. The far pencil should now be making a gateway, which is itself enclosed by the paired images of the reference point. Again, the paired images and the gateway should appear equally plain. Finally, focus somewhere in the middle distance, between the far pencil and the reference point, and see whether you can maintain not only both gateways but also the paired images of the reference point.

A more difficult two-pencil fusion involves focusing first on the near pencil, seeing the gateway made by the far pencil, dropping the near pencil from view, and then trying to maintain unchanged the gateway made by the far one. The same goes for dropping the far pencil and trying to maintain unchanged the paired reference point.

In another kind of pencil fusion the pencils are held side by side and a couple of inches apart. Use pencils of similar thickness but contrasting colour, say yellow and red. Holding the pencils at a convenient distance from your face, experiment until you are able to make of them a double gateway — that is, of three uprights, the central one consisting of the superimposed images of both pencils. Suppose the yellow pencil is in your left hand and the red in your right. Which colour is this central upright? If it is continuously of one colour — for example, red, corresponding to the colour seen by your stronger (right) eye — try to change it to yellow and back again to red, and then maintain it as a continuous superimposition of both colours.

Ruler fusion

In this the alignment of the visual axes is encouraged by the use of rulers of various lengths. If you are very myopic a short ruler — say 15 centimetres (6 inches) is easiest to begin with; aim to work up to a 30-centimetre (12-inch) ruler and ultimately to a metre rule (yardstick). Conversely, if you are very long-sighted or presbyopic, start with a long ruler and work down.

For the basic ruler fusion drill, hold the ruler edge-upwards and put one end between your eyes, so that one corner is resting on the bridge of your nose and the other on the lower part of your forehead. Hold the ruler from below, with the fingers of one hand, and align it so that it points straight out in front of you. If you now focus in the distance, the ruler should seem to be making a two-sided tunnel, both sides of which should be equally distinct. Practise bringing your focus back so that the far ends of the tunnel appear to approach each other and meet.

String fusion

For this you will need a piece of string between four and eight metres (13–26 feet) long. Thin white cord is best, but any sort of string will do. Tie a loop at one end to fit a nail or hook in the wall of your room, or over the door-handle or some other convenient projection. Then tie a knot every 30 centimetres (12 inches) or so along the string. Attach a small weight (such as an old key) to the end, to stop it from straying, and your fusion string is complete.

The projection over which you hook the loop should be roughly at eye level. Hold the string taut, with it touching the tip of your nose. Try to focus halfway along the string. If your fusion is already reasonably good, you should find that the string forms an X, with the crossover at the point you are looking at. As in all fusion work, both parts of the image (in this case "both" strings) ought to appear equally plain. If you cannot see the X, lower the string a little and try again, shutting your stronger eye if necessary, as in pencil fusion. If after this you still cannot see the X, give up string fusion for a while. It is more difficult than pencil or ruler fusion; but it is also one of the most valuable fusion techniques and you should plan to return to it later and try again.

On the other hand, if you do see the X, try focusing on one of the knots. Note the appearance of the X, and move to the next knot along. Eventually you should be able to move easily from knot to knot, back and forth along the whole length of the string, keeping the X going all the time.

Focus next on a point halfway between two knots. Making sure that both strings look equal, move your focus, slowly and with control, to one of the adjoining knots and back again to the midway point. Now move your focus to the other adjoining knot, and then to the middle of the next space along. Repeat with all the knots and spaces.

Picture fusion

The idea here is like that used in the drill with two differently coloured pencils. The images of the two objects are merged to make a third image.

Turn to Figure 10a, which shows two diagonal lines. Holding the page at a comfortable distance, vary the angle between your visual axes until you see not two objects, but three, the central one being a cross. Try holding the cross steady, with all four limbs of equal length. Figure 10b makes a triangle, 10c a cross inside a circle, 10d the same thing but with a smaller circle superimposed. In 10d, try to see the "crosshairs" inside the smaller circle. Figures 10e and 10f each produce two types of merged image; in 10f you should be able to see a pair of cartoon eyes, flanked by black dots. Turn the page sideways and upside-down to recombine the images in different ways.

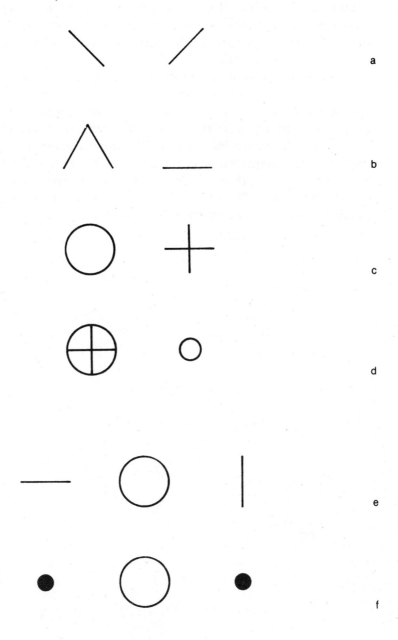

Figure 10: Fusion figures

Picture fusion is not easy, and if you have problems it may be helpful to use a ruler. A ruler — or batten of wood — with a non-shiny surface is to be preferred, as reflections can interfere with the correct perception of the fused image. Hold the ruler as in the basic drill, but place the far end on the page, between the two halves of the fusion picture. In this way you should be able to make them merge more readily.

The fusion pictures of Figure 10 are meant only as a suggestion: whether or not you have any drawing ability, it is more interesting to make your own. Any two images may be merged, provided their centres are not more than about five centimetres apart. Try drawing the outline of a face on one side, the features on the other, and then merge them; a monkey in a tree; a diver on a high board; a man and his hat, and so on. Or merge two real objects — buttons, coins, matchsticks. The greater the variety of the objects you use, the greater will be the benefit to your vision.

Mobility (I)

The techniques given under this heading, besides improving the remaining functions of the extrinsic muscles (tracking, searching, and scanning), also counteract the various tendencies which are part and parcel of the habit of "trying" to see. As already noted, this "trying" is commonly accompanied by some degree of immobility of the eyes and body. The rate of blinking decreases; breathing becomes shallower and may, for a while, even stop. The muscles of the head, neck, shoulders, and perhaps other parts of the body too, may be unnaturally tensed, and all the time the eyes are fixed with increasing intentness on their target. As the eyes become fixed so too does the attention, which only encourages the eyes to become yet more fixed, with a resulting impairment of both vision and perception.

Blinking and breathing

If you suspect yourself of staring in this way (and nearly everyone is prone to it), the first thing to do is to give thought to your blinking. Frequent, relaxed, and easy blinking is a requisite of good vision. The passage of the lids across the eyes lubricates the sclera where it is exposed to the air; the lachrymal fluid keeps the cornea clean; and, for several milliseconds at a time, light is excluded and the retina is rested. The lids also of course protect the eyes from injury, with a rapid reflex reaction to danger.

If proof were needed that there is a direct, demonstrable and intimate connection between the emotions and the physical workings of the eyes, it has been found that the rate of blinking varies with one's mental state. Blink-rate is used by behavioural scientists as a measure of attentiveness.

Practise giving half a dozen rapid and very light blinks, shut the eyes lightly for the space of two whole breaths, and repeat four times. This little routine, practised regularly, twice or more a day, will, especially if followed by a brief spell of palming, help to establish the correct tone in the muscles of the eyelids and develop better habits of blinking. No more than a few seconds should pass between one blink and the next. As a very rough guide, between two and four blinks in each period of ten seconds is about right.

Now and then throughout the day, whenever the idea occurs to you, take a moment to become aware of how often and how easily you are blinking. If you feel you are not blinking enough, deliberately increase your blink-rate a fraction and maintain this rate for as long as you can remember to.

Likewise, develop the art of occasional self-observation in your breathing. Whenever you catch yourself holding your breath as part of an attempt to see or to concentrate, issue a definite instruction to yourself to breathe freely. Do not try to interfere with your breathing mechanism, but simply take a few seconds in which to breathe easily and at the same time look about you, proving that there is after all no need to hold the breath in order to see.

Shifting

The fovea is that minute central region of the macula where the cones are most densely packed and resolution is best. At the centre of the fovea is a region smaller still, the foveola, where resolution reaches its limits. Correct use of the fovea relies on accurate scanning by the extrinsic muscles. When scanning is clumsy, the functional size of the foveola increases and its capacity to resolve the finest detail is lost. When scanning becomes yet worse, the differentiation in function between the fovea and the surrounding area of the macula is also lost.

The fovea is so small that only a tiny area of the visual field can be seen best at any given moment. The smaller the size of this area, the more precise the vision. It seems strange to think that we see best only when we see a tiny part of the visual field perfectly and the rest imperfectly; but that is exactly the case. In order for the brain to build up a detailed appreciation of any particular object in the visual field, this point of foveal vision must be scanned rapidly back and forth across the object, staying in one place for no more than a fraction of a second.

It is easy to discover whether your own scanning is working properly. Looking, for example, at the letter which begins this paragraph, if the uppermost tip is being regarded, then the rest of the letter should not be seen so well, and the bottom tip should be seen worst. If, at an ordinary reading distance, you find that you can see all parts of the letter, or even surrounding letters, equally well, then your scanning is poor: it is faulty in proportion to the size of the area on the page that you can see equally well all at once.

Scanning is an involuntary function of the extrinsic muscles, and so is quite unconscious and automatic. By consciously mimicking it, however, we can encourage, refine, and, if necessary, develop the mechanism whereby it is brought about, and this procedure is called "shifting".

For your preliminary exercise in shifting, place any one of the three test charts (Charts A, B, and C) where you can see it most clearly. Look first at the big C, and then shift your regard to the bottom line. You should now be aware that the C is not as clear as it was when you were looking straight at it. Shift back to the C, and then shift to the second line from the bottom, again acknowledging to yourself that the C has become less clear. Move up the chart in this way as far as you can. If you reach the second line down and the C still seems less clear, you are ready to move on to the next stage.

Start by shifting between the E and the L on the second line. Rather than thinking of the letter being regarded as the one seen *better*, think instead of the other one as being seen *worse*. This backwards sort of approach will help to prevent you from spoiling your vision by "trying" to see. Now move to the next line down, and shift between the O and the F and between the F and the S. Repeat with each line, shifting between each pair of letters. Remember to keep breathing normally. Rest the eyes at intervals with a little palming, and, as you palm, try shifting mentally between pairs of memorised letters.

The next stage is to shift between opposite corners of individual letters. E is a good one to begin with; L, H, F and V are also suitable. When you can shift between opposite corners on the letters of the bottom line, try shifting between, say, the middle and upper or the middle and lower bars of the letter E, or between the points of the letter U.

In future work, make your shifts as small and rapid as you can. Attempting shifts that are unnecessarily large or slow can cause strain. On the other hand, do not hurry to build up speed. Let it come gradually, of its own accord. Bear constantly in mind the fact that you have no targets to meet or opponents to overcome. Your progress will be very much an individual, idiosyncratic affair, and a competitive, striving attitude, in this as in all the practices of the Bates method, will only prove self-defeating.

Swinging

During shifting, the point of attention — the point where the two visual axes coincide — is constantly on the move, darting from point to point on the object being observed. The point of attention lies at the centre of the visual field, for it corresponds to the area perceived with the fovea. When the point of attention shifts, the whole visual field shifts with it, and the objects in view appear to shift accordingly.

If you now look away to the left of the page, the book should seem to move to the right, and if you look from side to side of, say, a picture on the far wall, it should appear to move back and forth in the opposite direction. The apparent movement of the book or picture, which is of course entirely illusory and relative, is called "swinging".

Swinging is the constant and natural accompaniment of foveal vision. When the eyesight is good, the swing is free and fluid, and is so much a part of normal perception that it is not usually remarked upon or even noticed. When viewed continuously, an object as small as a full stop on a page should appear to be making tiny pulsating swings corresponding to the scanning action of the eyes. The more rapid these movements and the smaller their range, the better the eyesight; as foveal vision deteriorates, so does the swing.

The swing can be encouraged, just as the scanning action can. However bad the eyesight, it should always be possible to produce some sort of swing, provided no undue effort is made to do so. By turning the head through 90 degrees or more, everyone should be able to recognise that the view seems to be moving past in the opposite direction. Practise making smaller and smaller swings, using the head at first and then the eyes alone.

Hold out your hand in front of you, palm downwards, at the distance where you see it best. Glance lightly at the outer edge of your thumb, and then glance immediately at the outer edge of your little finger. If your hand has swung, tuck your thumb out of sight, and glance from the edge of the little finger to the edge of the index finger. Repeat, reducing the number of fingers, until you can make your little finger swing on its own. Next, swing a pencil, a drinking straw, a darning needle, a pin.

Try also swinging individual letters on the test charts, beginning with the large letters and progressing to the smaller ones. Shift from side to side, from top to bottom, or from corner to corner, of each letter; or shift from a point a little way beyond the letter itself to the corresponding point on the opposite side, bringing the points closer until you can shift between points on the letter itself and still be aware of the swing.

Rest the eyes at intervals with palming, and as you do so visualise the letter you have just been looking at and continue to swing it mentally. When you open your eyes again, you may find that the swing of the real letter has become looser and freer.

Long swinging

There is another type of mobility swinging in the Bates method, sometimes called "long swinging", which has a rather different purpose. It is simple to do, and consists essentially of turning from side to side. Stand with the feet about 30 centimetres (12 inches) apart, the arms hanging loosely, and, lifting the right heel as you do so, turn to the left. When you have reached the limit of comfortable travel, turn to the right, letting the left heel rise and the right one return to the floor. Go on like this until you have performed 20 complete swings. The turning should involve your hips as well as your waist. Keep your arms relaxed so that they rise slightly as you swing. Do not go too fast: try to make the swings smooth, level, and rhythmical.

Keep your eyes open and allow the image of your surroundings to rush past without trying to focus on anything in particular. Nearby objects will naturally seem to move faster than distant ones; and will probably be no more than a blur. Make no attempt to hold on to or fix any part of the image; notice only that everything seems to be moving in the direction opposite to that of your swing.

Long swinging is very effective in breaking the habit of staring. It also promotes looseness and relaxation in the upper part of the body. According to Dr Bates, 50 swings performed at bedtime and again on rising will help to prevent or alleviate eyestrain during sleep.

Should you find yourself becoming dizzy, begin with just a few swings and each day add one or two to the total. Eventually any feeling of nausea should disappear and you will be able to do as many swings as you please.

Once you are proficient at full-travel swings, gradually reduce the travel until you are moving no more than 30 centimetres (one foot) from side to side. Stand in front of a window with an upright glazing bar, and find some vertical object in the view outside (a lamp-post, a tree, the side of a building). Now as you swing, notice that the glazing bar and the lamp-post or whatever seem to be moving in opposite directions. Observe this movement half a dozen times and then, still swinging, close the eyes. Visualise the movement during a few swings, and on opening your eyes see how your visualisation compared with the real thing. Close the eyes again and repeat. (If you do not have a window with a vertical glazing bar, hang a length of string from the frame or ceiling.)

In all swinging, continue to remember not to fix your eyes on any one part of the image. Become aware of the freedom and fluidity of your movement and the corresponding freedom and fluidity of the world beyond. As the head or eyes move, you will realise that your normal relationship with objects in view has been subtly changed. Now that you have been relieved, as it were, of the necessity of fixing your eyes on the world in order to give it existence, you will find that it continues to exist none the less.

Carry the awareness of this over into everyday life. As you move about indoors, walk along the street or through the woods, ride a bike, travel about by bus, train, or car, try to become conscious of the constant movement in the view, and of the relative speed of objects both far and near. Notice how the speed of movement imparts a greater sense of depth and reality to the scene. Our visual system has evolved in a world of three dimensions, a world of constant movement and change. An appreciation of this is one of the most important steps towards restoring the mobility of attention on which good eyesight depends.

Mobility (II)

It should be said that direct attempts to improve foveal vision by consciously shifting can sometimes prove difficult at first. You may find it better to postpone practice of conscious shifting for a while and concentrate instead on the techniques in this chapter, which are both a practical expression of foveal vision and a means of encouraging it. When your foveal vision has been improved by these indirect means, they can be used in conjunction with direct shifting and swinging to improve it yet further.

The following techniques all involve the idea of getting the eyes and mind to work together, either by searching the visual field or by following objects in motion. They are offered mainly by way of suggestion. You can doubtless think of many more yourself.

The first are based on the sort of pastimes that, before the advent of television, used to keep children (and not a few adults) amused on wet afternoons.

Dominoes

Dominoes are an ideal object on which to practise foveal vision. There is good contrast between the black background and the white or coloured dots, and, in order to identify each stone, the eye must make a series of rapid shifts. The game of dominoes in all its variants provides an entertaining source of practice, if you enjoy playing; but, even if you don't, the dominoes themselves may be put to good use as an aid to vision.

Take a set of dominoes and arrange them in random rows and columns, such as those shown in Figure 11. Either wedge the stones into a shallow box lid or glue them (double sided adhesive tape is handy for this) to a piece of stout, and preferably red, cardboard.

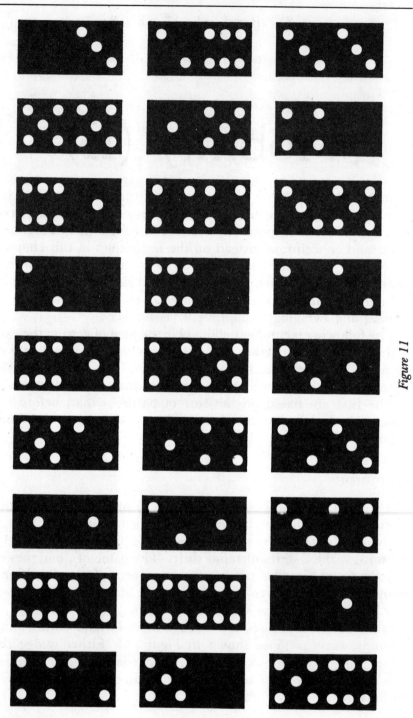

Figure 11

Place the dominoes just inside your "blur zone" — that is, just out of focus. Palm for half a minute, and then look along each row of half-stones, starting at the top left-hand corner, moving from left to right, dropping one row, coming back from right to left, dropping to the next row, and so on. Thus the sequence in the example of Figure 11 would be 4-6-1-5-6-2-6-5-0-3-5-1-0-3-2-1-4-2-5- etc. Speak each number to yourself and rapidly move on to the next. Do not worry if you make a mistake. What matters is the attempt to count the dots and the rapid movement on to the next group. Close the eyes for a moment or two at the end of each row. Repeat, but this time name the numbers in the columns rather than the rows. Vary the practice further by finding each number in sequence, or by finding each domino in ascending or descending order of value, or by subtracting the value of one half-stone from its neighbour and finding the product elsewhere — any sort of arithmetical operation can be pressed into service to make the drill more interesting.

At subsequent sessions, move the dominoes slightly deeper into your blur zone, but remember never to strain or to try too hard to count the dots. If you don't have any real dominoes to hand, Figure 11 itself may be used instead.

The use of dominoes like this has been found specially helpful in cases of astigmatism, for which the following drill may also be of use.

Bring the dominoes to within 7–10 centimetres (3–4 inches) of your face and move them fairly quickly from side to side, back and forth in front of your eyes, 10 or 20 times, moving the dominoes so that new rows of dots are being presented at each pass. As the dominoes move to the left, turn your head a little to the right, and vice versa. Next, turn the board or box lid the other way round and pass the dominoes before your eyes from top to bottom rather than from side to side, again between 10 and 20 times, and again presenting fresh rows of dots at each pass. It will be seen that this technique has something in common with long swinging; and, as in long swinging, no attempt should be made to focus on or hold any part of the image. Be content to see the dots as a continuous blurred stream against the black background of the stones.

Dice and other games

Like dominoes, dice are easy to see and require the eyes to make a number of shifts while the brain is counting. They are equally useful for encouraging mobility and, as they are so small, may easily be carried about in the purse or pocket for use in odd moments.

Throw your dice by hand rather than with a canister. As they come to rest, take a very rapid glance at the upper faces and immediately close your eyes. Visualise the dice and the way they have fallen, and name the value of each one. Briefly look back at them to compare your visualisation with the real thing. Here again, accuracy is less important than the act of getting your eyes and mind to move. Repeat several times.

Start with just two dice, and slowly work up to four or even five. Small dice are better than large ones. Once you are able to visualise all the upper faces, try visualising some of the other faces too, first on the left hand side of one die, then on both sides, and then on more than one die. When you throw the dice, try not to spread them too widely.

Any game which makes use of dice, from snakes and ladders to backgammon, gives excellent practice in shifting. So too do such games as chess, chequers, snooker, and, best of all, Scrabble, in which one must continuously search the board or table for new combinations. Certain fast-moving computer games, especially when viewed on a monitor rather than a domestic television set, are also good, as are the pocket-sized electronic games which have a liquid crystal display and use beeps to engage the hearing as well as the eyesight.

Playing-cards also provide an opportunity for entertainment combined with exercise in shifting. For their value in this, though, the various games must be reassessed according to their speed, so that snap and cheat come out at the top of the list, and bridge and poker at the bottom. One of the best games for our purposes is patience, particularly the variety in which the cards are laid out in seven columns. Acquire if you can a pack of miniature cards and use these in preference to the ordinary ones, especially if you already see fairly well at reading distance.

Ball games of any kind are good for mobility, whether played or watched. The smaller the ball and the faster it moves and changes direction the better. Indeed, the projectile need not be a ball—it can be a shuttlecock, a frisbee, or even a boomerang: the effect is the same. Two-ball juggling is a valuable exercise. Toss one ball with your left hand and catch it with your right, and, while it is in the air, *throw* the other ball from your right hand to your left. Keep the balls moving inside an imaginary box, and make sure your eyes follow the left-hand ball throughout its trajectory. Juggling like this outdoors, gradually turning so that you approach the brightest part of the sky, is effective too in helping to overcome photophobia.

Random numbers

The table of random numbers (see Appendix B) contains each of the numbers from 1 to 99, printed at least once. By searching the table for combinations or sequences of numbers, the attention is encouraged to shift very rapidly indeed.

With the table at your normal reading distance (or as close as you can bring it if you are hypermetropic or presbyopic), search for the numbers from 1 to 50. That will probably be enough for your first session. On subsequent days, search for some other sequence: 50 to 99, perhaps, or 99 to 30, or whatever you choose. As you become familiar with the table you will remember where certain numbers are to be found; to minimise this effect, at alternate sessions search by column or by row, and gradually increase the length of the search sequence so that eventually you go from 1 to 99 and back again to 1. The search may be varied in other ways. Pick a pair of numbers at random—say 93 and 04. Take the first digit from the first and the second from the second to form a new number, in this case 94, which you then proceed to find in the table. Having found 94, pair it with an adjacent number in the same way and find the next. Other sorts of combinations, involving addition, subtraction, multiplication, division, people's birthdays or telephone numbers, etc., can of course be sought as well.

The number board

Fix the number board (Chart D), at a distance where the largest grid of numbers is easily legible, the middle-sized one less so, and the smallest is legible only with difficulty. Make yourself comfortable, palm for a minute or so, and, on opening your eyes, glance at the largest 1. Holding the memory of the figure, close your eyes and, breathing freely and normally, turn your head to the right until your chin is roughly in line with your shoulder. Open your eyes, let the 1 go and, not too quickly, turn back. Glance now at the largest 2; close the eyes and turn to the left. Continue swinging slowly and rhythmically in this way until you become tired or have covered all the numbers up to 20. As you approach each number, let your gaze travel in the blank spaces under the line of numbers rather than across the numbers themselves, so that when you come to the appointed figure you make a slight upwards shift.

In the next stage, repeat the process, except that, when you glance at each of the numbers on the largest grid, glance immediately to the left and find its medium-sized counterpart. When you close your eyes, hold the memory of the medium-sized figure, giving to it, however, the clarity of your perception of the largest figure.

Repeat the drill once more, but this time find, with a rapid, unconcerned glance, the smallest figure as well. You will know its position on the grid, but it is not important whether you are conscious of perceiving the figure in any detail. Merely close your eyes and hold in your mind the image of what you *did* see, while lending to it the clearer memory of the largest figure.

Reading

The act of recognising a single letter requires the eye to perform at least one shift and probably more. While reading, it is the shapes of words which tend to be recognised rather than their component letters, but nonetheless a large number of shifts — perhaps several dozen — must be performed in order to read a sentence. Reading a whole chapter will demand many thousands of shifts, and for this reason reading is excellent for encouraging mobility.

The matter read should first of all be of interest, and the print should if possible be small rather than large, because then the range of each shift will also be small. The abnormally large print, supposed to be easier to read, used in children's books actually does the children no favour at all. Because the letters are so large, the child's eye must perform abnormally large shifts in order to take in the shapes of letters and words, thus postponing or even interfering with the acquisition of the correct visual habits necessary for reading print of ordinary size.

For our purposes, the smaller the print the better, provided there is adequate space between each line. Small print with generous spaces between the lines is always more legible than large print with narrow spaces.

Let the eye run just below the line of letters, for this discourages the tendency to "catch hold" of any part of the sentence. At first it may feel strange, but if you persevere you should find that reading becomes much easier.

For those who have trouble focusing at reading distance, it often helps actually to isolate the sentences from each other, so that you can be sure of reading them one at a time. Take a sheet of stiff paper about 15 centimetres (6 inches) square (black paper is best as it improves contrast), and, using a razor-sharp blade and a straight edge, cut a slot across the middle just over 10 centimetres (4 inches) wide and 5 millimetres (3/16 inch) high. This size is about right for most novels and similarly printed books; for material in other formats, papers with appropriately sized slots should be prepared, or, with a little ingenuity, an adjustable slot can be made. Failing that, simply place a 12-centimetre (5-inch) strip of paper or thin card under each line of type and move it down the page as you read.

Isolating the lines like this prevents neighbouring lines from jostling for your attention. In some cases it is worth going one stage further: make the slot of the same height but no more than about 2.5 centimetres (1 inch) wide, enabling only one or two words to be seen at a time. Move the slot along the line as you read.

All reading and close work generally should be done under strong illumination. Not only will a strong light improve the contrast between the print and the blank paper, but it will also encourage foveal vision and stop down the iris to increase the depth of focus. Using a slot and under a bright lamp, you may find it possible to read print which formerly was beyond you.

Take frequent breaks during your reading to make use of the other techniques of the method. Palming, visualisation, and sunning are especially helpful in preventing or alleviating the eyestrain and headaches that often accompany or follow reading.

Edging

This little technique is one of the most effective there is for normalising and coordinating the various functions of the extrinsic muscles. It may be practised virtually anywhere and at any time. All that is needed is an object in view with a definite and easily perceived edge — a picture rail, a door frame, a book on the table, telephone wires, the rise of a hillside.

Follow the edge, whatever it is, with your eyes. In the case of a picture frame, you might start at the top left-hand corner and edge each side in turn, moving clockwise, and then retrace your path, ending where you started. Or you might edge the picture frame several times in one direction, and then several times in the other. Give preference to objects in your blur zone, but do not neglect to edge other objects too.

The effects of edging are enhanced if, at the same time, you look down the "tunnel" described in the section on ruler fusion (p. 55).

Observation

Perhaps the best — because the most natural — way to get your foveal vision working properly is to cultivate the habit of being observant. Many people seem to pass through life in a sort of haze, never actually seeing anything they look at. The converse of this state, perpetual alertness, is very difficult, if not impossible, to achieve; but at least it gives us a goal to work towards.

Trained observers do their seeing in response to a continuous flow of unconscious questions. If the observer is a policeman, say, the questions will be of the type likely to be put to him at some future date in court; if he is a scientist, they might be those that critical colleagues would ask in order to verify whatever it is he is trying to prove. In any event, the questions asked are of just a few fundamental sorts: "How many? What size, shape, colour? What special features — what similarities and differences?"

Teach yourself to ask these questions, consciously at first, about whatever is in view. To start with you might, whenever you think of it, apply the question "How many?" to the view. "How many people at the bus stop? How many windows in that house? How many panes in each window?" If the numbers are large, your counting need not be more than approximate — all that really matters is that you are getting your eyes and mind to move and work together.

Later, when you have become proficient at each type of observation in turn, combine one type with another, and then with two others, and with others yet, until you can combine them all simultaneously and it becomes second nature to see observantly. If you are looking at a vase of flowers, for instance, you will no longer be satisfied to look at it without seeing. You will want to know at least one fact about it and probably more. How many flowers? What species? What colours? Is there anything unusual about them? What of the vase itself? Is it glazed or not, plain or decorated? Have you ever seen one like it before?

This all sounds like rather hard work, but in fact an analytical observation of our vase of flowers would take no more than a couple of moments and would be performed quite automatically. This, after all, is the way our eyes were meant to be used. For primitive man, survival itself depended on a keen and constant appreciation of detail and change. The slightest clue — a pawprint, a broken twig — might be the only warning he had of hidden danger. Civilisation has removed the need for such vigilance, but it has also blunted our senses and deprived us of the pleasure of being properly aware of our surroundings.

As with a number of practices in the Bates method, the effects of analytical observation may be heightened with the use of mental imagery. Using the technique just described, and, to begin with, at the distance at which you see it best, study an object or group of objects, shut your eyes, and examine closely the image that remains. When you feel you have recalled as much as you can, open your eyes and compare the real with the recollected image. Close them again and repeat several times.

Each time you repeat the process you will take in more information, steadily improving your knowledge of whatever you are looking at. The final images (real as well as recalled) should be considerably more vivid and detailed than the first.

The benefits of this practice will accrue as a livelier, more interested approach to observation and seeing generally, and as a gradual improvement in and development of the visual memory. This in turn will benefit the ability to perceive rapidly and well.

Accommodation

Whatever the truth about the mechanism of accommodation, there can be little doubt that it is based on muscular movement or something very much like it. Regular use and exercise of muscle systems elsewhere in the body always lead towards health and normality of function, and there is no reason to suppose that the same is not true of the muscle systems of the eye.

Let us once again go back to first principles, and consider the way the human species has evolved. Until a very recent time, in evolutionary terms, that is, the human animal made its shelters of brushwood and skins, or took refuge in those rather rare but secure natural shelters, caves. Because artificial lighting was so primitive as to be almost useless, the shelters were occupied mainly for sleeping or during bad weather. For the rest of the time, our ancestors spent their lives outdoors, whether hunting, fishing, gathering food plants, making or repairing clothes or utensils, or just sitting round the camp fire doing nothing. They spent their lives outdoors, because there were no such things as doors.

The point is that the human eye evolved in conditions very different from those that prevail today. The universal use of electric lighting, and the simple fact that we now live in buildings, have together deprived the eye of distance and severely limited the range over which most of its accommodation is done. It is noteworthy that glasses are unusual among those people — agricultural workers, for example — whose way of life demands that they spend much of their time under the sky.

Once any muscle is deprived of its full and normal range of use, it begins to atrophy. So with the mechanism of accommodation. Lack of distance — together with the emotional causes discussed in previous chapters—is one of the factors contributing to its deterioration. If the other causes are overcome, if glasses are not worn, and if the eye is again supplied with the full range of distance it needs, focusing ability will gradually be restored.

What this means in practical terms is that you should endeavour to get out and about at least once a day; and, when you are out, let your eye range constantly from far to near. This will help you whether you are long-sighted or short-sighted, but short-sighted people will find it of special benefit. Make the most of bright, sunny days, because then the pupil contracts, the depth of focus is increased, and refractive error is reduced to its minimum, so that the eye is more likely to be coaxed into better habits of accommodation. For developing better eyesight, walking is the way to travel, as then you have time to appreciate the view as well as the depth of field as made manifest by passing objects. Do not waste any opportunities for distance vision afforded by trips by road or rail, although looking through glass is never as satisfactory as being in the open air.

You can encourage the recovery of focusing ability by allowing the eye to follow approaching or departing vehicles. Car number-plates or the lettering on vans and lorries may be used as convenient "test charts", and any journey by road can be transformed into a session of accommodation practice. Even better than this is to stand on a bridge over a motorway; if you are long-sighted, concentrate on watching the traffic as it approaches and passes below you; if you are short-sighted, allow the receding vehicles to draw your gaze ever further into the distance. Watch one vehicle at a time, and memorise brief episodes from this practice for use later in your palming and visualisation sessions. It does not matter if your focusing ability does not keep pace with your attention. One of the causes of difficulty in accommodation is a subconscious reluctance to look into the distance or close to, and the mere fact that you are deliberately challenging this reluctance is enough to bring about an improvement in attitude and hence, ultimately, in accommodation itself.

When indoors you should remain aware of the need for frequent changes of focus. While reading, look up from the page at regular intervals—say at the end of each long paragraph or each page—and, just for a second, consciously focus on some distant object. While watching television, keep a light on in the room and frequently look away from the screen, whether at an object nearer or farther away.

If you are already able to focus at reading distance, get into the habit of, now and then when you are alone, examining very closely some small object. Insects — if you can bring yourself to look at them — make a fascinating subject for study with the naked eye, as do leaves, flowers, bits of bark, ferns, feathers, pebbles: in fact, anything from nature. Examine also the minute appearance and texture of such objects as your front door key, pen nib, or wristwatch. Use both eyes together, and from time to time measure and make a note of the minimum distance at which you are able to focus.

Besides these suggestions for accommodation practice in day to day life, the Bates method provides certain specific drills, each of which is a variation on the same theme of exercising the mechanism of accommodation.

Zooming

This is perhaps the simplest of the accommodation drills. Cut a strip of paper about eight centimetres (three inches) long and two centimetres (slightly under an inch) wide, and in the centre mark a small ink cross. Wrap the strip of paper round the base of the middle finger of your left hand, in such a way that the cross is towards you when the palm is uppermost. The strip is held in place by your ring and index fingers.

Cover your right eye with your right hand and, watching the cross, bring it slowly closer, and closer still, beyond your nearpoint, until it is merely a blur, and then make it slowly retreat. Take it out to arm's length and bring it back rather more quickly. Do this five times in all, accelerating as you go, so that at the end your hand is moving fairly rapidly.

Repeat with the right hand and the right eye, and then, still with the strip on your right hand, with both eyes together. Pause, look into the distance, and repeat the whole drill once more. Slowly build up to five repetitions, making six sets in all. Zooming can be relatively strenuous in the beginning, so do not try to attempt too much, and stop immediately if you find yourself becoming tired or losing interest. Should you not have a bit of paper by you, close your hand slightly so that one of the creases in your palm becomes more pronounced, and use that as your object instead.

Using the test charts

The basic test chart (Chart A) comes with two reductions of itself at one quarter and one eighth scale (Charts B and C). Depending on the nature of your refractive error and the state of your eyesight, you should be able to read part of at least two of the charts when the larger is at the distance and the smaller is near at hand. By "the distance" is meant any distance in excess of 3 metres (10 feet) and, for practical purposes, under about 6 metres (20 feet). If you are very myopic or your sight is otherwise bad, "the distance" may be taken to mean the greatest range at which you can read the first two or three lines of Chart A. For some, that may be as near as a couple of metres (5 to 6 feet). As your Bates training proceeds, you should be able to increase this fairly steadily until you can read two or more lines of Chart A at 3 metres (10 feet).

Fix Chart A to the wall at eye level. You may find it convenient to paste the chart to a sheet of hardboard or stout card and arrange a loop of string at the back, picture-fashion, so that it can be taken down when not required. Make sure the chart is in a good light. Strong daylight is best. The standard specification for opticians' test charts recommends two ordinary 60 watt lamps mounted about 35 centimetres (15 inches) from the chart and inclined towards it at an angle of about 15 degrees, or a single 100 watt spotlight reflector (of the type mentioned in the chapter on sunning) about 1.5 metres (5 feet) away. This level of illumination is adequate for testing, but for visual re-education a considerably brighter light is better. If the 100 watt spotlight is brought to within 50 centimetres (20 inches) of the chart or less, the pupil of the eye contracts and depth of focus is improved. This level is recommended for all practice work with the chart, number board, dominoes, and any other material at the distance.

Now, seated at a table or in a comfortable chair, prop or hold one of the smaller charts in front of you, in such a way that you can glance easily from one chart to the other. If you can read Chart C, use that; otherwise use Chart B. In either case the apparent size of the small chart should be about the same as that of Chart A. The small chart, like Chart A, should be strongly illuminated, preferably to a similar level, so that the two charts resemble each other in all respects but their distance from your eyes.

Palm for a while, and then look at the chart which you see more clearly. Starting with the big C, and continuing with each letter in turn, find the letter first on this chart and then on the other one. Notice that the letters are identical in everything but distance. The letters are inert, waiting to be seen. They are made of printers' ink, one of the blackest substances known. The reason that you see the letters of one chart grey and the other black has nothing to do with the letters themselves. The illusion lies entirely in your own perception. The grey letters are every bit as black as the others. As you look at them, acknowledge this self-evident fact to yourself, and, without reference to what you are actually seeing, imagine that they appear just as black as the letters on the easier chart. Try also the same visualisation technique as you used with the number board, assigning to the imperfectly seen letter the blackness and clarity of the other.

Read as much as you can (without strain) of the easy chart, palm once more, and repeat the whole process. If you are able to read part or all of Chart C at reading distance, vary the procedure on occasion by having all three charts in view and looking from one to another in ascending or descending order of size.

The test charts, singly or together, may be used in other ways also. The letters serve as excellent subjects for visualisation, swinging, and shifting. Practise shifting from top to bottom and side to side of individual letters, first on the easier chart and then on the harder one. Shift also between similar letters of different sizes on the same chart. Then shift between corresponding pairs of letters on the other chart. As you transfer your glance from far to near, do so easily and unconcernedly. Remember always that good vision cannot be achieved through effort or strain.

As a supplement to the charts, an astigmatism indicator is provided in Appendix B. According to the nature of your astigmatism, if you have any, at least one of the arms of the indicator will appear more blurred than the others.

The charts and the indicator are invaluable in reinforcing the feedback from brain to eye. This feedback is the key to recovering focusing ability. If the image improves, however fleetingly, the brain needs to be informed and, as it were, congratulated. It must be encouraged to repeat whatever it did that produced the improvement. The letters on a test chart, unlike most ordinary objects, give a very precise indication of how well the eyes are working. Looking at a chart between spells of palming will alert you to any changes, no matter how subtle, that are taking place in your vision. At first these changes will be so slight that you will probably dismiss them as imaginary — until, perhaps, you recall that imagination and vision are very much of the same. Later the changes will become more marked and dramatic, and you will almost certainly be surprised to find how much your eyesight varies from moment to moment and from day to day.

Vision
and the Mind

It has been repeatedly emphasised so far that vision is a function
not only of the eyes, but of the mind as well. This attitude marks
the fundamental difference in approach between orthodox
ophthalmologists and teachers of the Bates method. Opticians seem
content to treat the eyes as though they are somehow independent
of the brain; as though they are mere optical instruments whose
performance, if lacking, can be restored by means of auxiliary
lenses.

The Bates teacher holds such a view to be mistaken. He holds
that the relationship between the eyes and the mind that controls
them is just as subtle and complicated as the mind itself. Already
we have seen how the method enlists the aid of such allies of vision
as imagination and memory, and how, through cultivating a
certain mental approach, we can help to improve the conditions
under which vision takes place. We will now explore a little more
deeply the relationship between eyes and mind, with a view to
improving these conditions yet more.

Unconscious vision

An early consequence of beginning Bates training is an increased
awareness of how well or badly one's eyesight is working. One
becomes more sensitive to its performance and more alive to
sensations that formerly, when wearing glasses, one would have

missed. This is particularly true when it comes to the phenomenon of unconscious vision.

This term is here applied to that part of the visual process which is completed before the conscious mind becomes involved. When you look at something, the information from the retina is developed to quite a high level before being routed into the conscious part of the visual process. It is obvious that, even if the rest of the visual system is operating normally, there can be no perception until the conscious mind is prepared to accept the incoming information.

According to the Bates hypothesis, faulty vision can arise as one result of emotional difficulties, among which may be a subsconscious desire not to see. As far as refractive error is concerned, this desire not to see can be compared to the desire not to walk or talk shown in certain kinds of hysterical illness. The brain is able to block the responses of the body so that walking or talking — or focusing — do indeed become more difficult, or even impossible.

The brain can also block the visual process in another way, by erecting a barrier of some sort between the unconscious and the conscious mind, so that, even if the eyes are performing well, the signals are obstructed or degraded before being allowed to reach the consciousness.

It is helpful to think of this barrier in symbolic terms, as being made of some substance which can vary in consistency according to the subconscious wishes of the brain. When vision is perfect the substance of the barrier is perfectly fluid and the signals pass through it freely, but as vision deteriorates the substance becomes more and more glutinous, slowing down the passage of the signals or preventing it altogether.

Thus there are two distinct ways in which the brain can block the visual process. The first is by interfering with the mechanics of vision; the second is by altering the "consistency" of the barrier between the unconscious and the conscious mind.

The first type of blocking tends to succumb more readily to the techniques of the Bates method. After a few weeks of Bates training, one often begins to experience clear flashes — fleeting moments of perfect or near-perfect eyesight. The clear flashes come when the eyes and mind are working together, unimpeded by the conscious self which tries to see or in other ways interferes with vision, and unimpeded by any subconscious desire not to see. To begin with, the excitement and astonishment caused by the clear flashes usually engages the conscious mind again, the bad habits instantly return, and so the clear flash instantly disappears. A clear flash can be so brief that one cannot be sure that it really took place, although one is left with a feeling that something has in fact happened. During clear flashes, then, both types of blocking are temporarily absent.

Because the first type of blocking tends to be less difficult to overcome than the second, there will be moments when the eyes are working in an improved way but their signals are prevented from passing through the barrier. Such moments give rise to the phenomenon of unconscious vision — when information is in the visual system but is not recognised for what it is.

To give an example from my own experience, I remember walking towards a car parked a good distance along the road. As I approached it I somehow knew what two letters of the numberplate were, even though the whole sequence was as yet a myopic blur. To my surprise I found that I had been right about the two letters, and almost right about a third — for I had imagined it to be an O and it turned out to be a D. My eyes must have been working perfectly for the instant it took them to scan the first two letters, but, by the time they came to the third, they had already started to lose focus. The information about the three letters — positive identification of the first two, and a vague feeling about the third — was transmitted to my brain and expressed there in sub-visual terms, that is, as an intuition.

It could well be argued that I might have seen the car and its numberplate before and remembered the letters. That is entirely possible, but the same thing happened not just once, but often, in unfamiliar as well as familiar places, and with a variety of lettering and numerals besides car numberplates.

Flashing

In the example just given, I had seen more than I thought I had. During practice of the Bates method, one soon comes to realise that this is a frequent — perhaps even the usual — state of affairs. If a guess is made about something, especially if the guess is made in a spirit of confident indifference as to its correctness, then it very often turns out that the guess is right. Guessing, after all, is the essence of perception: we opt for the most likely solution, based on probability and past experience. Perception is really nothing more than a series of educated guesses.

Freeing the barrier between the unconscious and the conscious mind can be accelerated by encouraging this guessing process. Take a rapid glance at something in your blur zone — a domino, for example, or a playing-card. Close your eyes and then, without caring too much whether you are right or wrong, make a guess about the number of dots or the identity of the card. If your answer is even partly right you will be ahead; if it is completely wrong, you will be no worse off than you were before.

It is essential to acknowledge that there is nothing wrong or dishonest about guessing like this. Indeed, the opposite approach — a disinclination to trust oneself, a reliance only on what one is sure of seeing — is wrong because it goes contrary to the way that perception works.

The procedure of taking a rapid glance and then a guess about what has been seen is called, in the Bates method, "flashing". It may be practised during daily life whenever you have the opportunity, using such objects as street-signs, numberplates, and advertising hoardings. It may also be practised during special drills. Depending on whether you see better at the distance or near to, try flashing dominoes or playing-cards held at arm's length or set up a few metres away. If you can find an assistant, flash playing-cards drawn at random from the pack, shown to you for a moment and then replaced. Similar drills can easily be devised using Scrabble or mahjong tiles, dice, photos or advertisements cut from magazines, etc.

Familiarisation

If perception consists of a series of educated guesses, we can state as a corollary that something familiar will be easier to see than something new. That is why the experienced naturalist sees things in the countryside that are invisible to anyone else. He notices a certain sort of bird in a tree because he has seen one many times before and so has been educated in knowing where to look and what to look for. His threshold of recognition has been lowered by familiarity. The same is true of anyone who has special knowledge and recollection of what to look for in his surroundings.

It is clearly an advantage to be as familiar as possible with your environment. If you develop the habit of analytical observation such familiarity will come anyway, but it helps to make a special study of those objects and features that are most important to us and most often seen. The faces of family and friends, for example, should be studied in detail and facts about them remembered; the same goes for the structure and contents of the rooms where you live and work, the vehicles you habitually use, and so on.

You may already believe that you are thoroughly familiar with some of the most important and commonly encountered objects of all — the objects you are looking at now. Quite frequently, though, when the vision is defective, it has been found that there is only a partial appreciation of the exact form of many of the letters of the alphabet, especially when they are printed in lower case rather than capitals. Both to make reading easier and as a curious little exercise for its own sake, try examining each letter in turn, in a variety of different sizes and styles, upside-down and sideways as well as the right way up. Observe and remember the shapes and angles, not only of the letter itself but also of the white spaces surrounding or enclosed by it. Notice how certain letters are sometimes combined in ligatures or diphthongs such as ff, ffi, and æ. By comparing individual letters in upper and lower case and in different styles — with or without serifs, plain, italic, bold, Old English, Saxon, shadow, and so on — try to decide what it is that gives each letter its own unique identity. What is the essential pattern that the typeface designer must preserve in order for the letter to remain recognisable? Do the same with the ten numerals, punctuation marks, and other common symbols such as ½, %, @, *, &.

Since familiar objects are easier to see, it is suggested that, before using the test charts, especially when one is used on its own and at a distance where some of the letters look blurred, you should acquaint yourself thoroughly with each line and memorise its sequence.

Until you are comfortably familiar with the layout of the charts, use the number board for any work in your blur zone.

More visualisation techniques

These, like the ones described in earlier chapters, help to reinforce and coordinate the relationship between memory, imagination, and vision.

The first follows on from the ideas presented in the sections on palming and shifting. While looking at a letter on the test chart, imagine a small spot of deeper black, like a full stop, on one corner of the letter. The full stop should be as small as possible, but at first you may find it easier to imagine a larger spot of black and at subsequent sessions progressively reduce its size. Shift to the opposite corner of the letter and imagine the full stop there. As you shift, become conscious of the swing. Having repeated this several times with the eyes open, palm and continue to do it with your mind's eye, still remaining conscious of the swing. Open the eyes again and repeat.

It will be realised that here we are using the imagination and memory to mimic the effects of foveal vision, for when the eyesight is good the point being regarded on a letter always appears blacker than the rest.

To take this practice one stage further, imagine while palming three dots printed in a row. Shift from one to another at random, seeing worse the two you are not looking at. The swing in this case will be manifested as an apparent movement of the line of dots to left or right. Imagine that the dots are of an extremely intense black; picture yourself making them with the tip of a fine brush impregnated with Indian ink. The paper is as intensely white as the dots are black. After a little while, tear off that sheet of paper and throw it away. Make three new dots, even finer than the others and more closely spaced. Repeat, being as extravagant as you like with your imaginary pad, until the dots are as fine and black as you can make them.

On the next occasion, take a tiny and imaginary pair of compasses and in Indian ink scribe a small circle. Just above it and to either side, mark a small dot with the compass pen. Shift between the two dots and note how the circle appears to swing. On another day, mark the paper with a colon and a semicolon side by side and shift between the quartet of marks, noting again how the swing behaves, and seeing worse the marks you are not looking at.

Again with your imaginary pad, imagine that your nose has somehow become prolonged into a paintbrush or pen loaded with the blackest of black inks. Draw a square on the paper, accompanying the imaginary movements of your head with real ones. Your control will not be so accurate as when drawing in the ordinary way, so go over each line a few times until you are reasonably happy with the result. Now tear off that sheet and draw a large circle. Draw another just inside it, and a small one at the centre, like the hub of a cartwheel. Then draw the spokes radiating from the hub to the rim. Taking a fresh sheet, and changing if you feel like it your brush for a pen or vice versa, try drawing something else a little more ambitious, or else sign your name or write a phrase.

This nose-writing technique may sound rather ludicrous, but it has proved invaluable in breaking the habit of staring. It may also be adapted for use with the eyes open. When you are talking on the telephone, for example, give your eyes something to do: follow the tip of your pen as you write or doodle.

It should be mentioned here that it is not good to allow the eyes to stare vacantly into space, as most of us are apt to do when daydreaming. The eyes are meant to be used. If you temporarily have no work for them, close the lids and give your visual system a rest.

Attitudes to seeing

It can hardly be repeated too often that cultivating the right attitude towards seeing is a vital part of the process of re-education. With a negative, pessimistic attitude, no progress is possible; but, conversely, too much optimism can be a bad thing, for it usually leads to disappointment.

A useful analogy can be drawn if we compare seeing with another complex function, the sense of balance. Anyone can walk along a rope if it is laid along the carpet, but only an expert can do the same thing five or ten or fifty metres up. Why? The answer is obvious: the ordinary person is afraid of falling. He has no confidence in his ability to prevent himself from falling, and his fear dominates his sense of balance. The fear becomes a conviction, and so, not surprisingly, he falls.

Something essentially similar, if less dramatic, happens when the eyesight begins to deteriorate. Having once been unable to focus correctly on a given object in a given set of circumstances, we naturally fear that we will be unable to focus correctly next time. The fear is father to the conviction, and the conviction dominates the subtle act of accommodation. The result is that our fear and conviction are confirmed, making it even harder to focus in the future. So it goes on, a vicious circle leading to the stage where any possibility of focusing correctly is out of the question.

During the whole of your Bates training you should try to maintain a jaunty indifference to the success or failure of your efforts. If at any moment you cannot see a given object, even though perhaps yesterday or just now you could, *it does not matter*. The short term is not important. Your refractive error probably took a long time to develop, and you are unlikely to get rid of it overnight. Once you have satisfied yourself that your eyesight is variable and can, by means of the Bates method, be varied for the better, then the foundation of the right attitude towards your progress will have been laid.

CHAPTER
NINE

The Method
in Practice

We have now looked at all the techniques of the Bates method. As already mentioned, you should experiment with each to find out which ones suit you best. You ought to be able to find at least one or two, and perhaps more, from each of the five main categories — palming, sunning, fusion, mobility, and accommodation. This selection will then form the basis of your initial approach to the method.

The techniques are nearly all of application in every case of defective eyesight. In some, such as visualisation or the accommodation drills, the emphasis is varied according to the kind of difficulty which it is desired to overcome; and the following are likely to be of particular benefit for specific problems:

Myopia — palming with visualisation, analytical observation, spending time outdoors;

Hypermetropia — long swinging, zooming;

Presbyopia — simple palming;

Astigmatism — all mobility techniques, especially dominoes, dice, etc., and edging.

The following may also be of special help in dealing with these other defects:

Floaters — sunning;

Squint — all fusion techniques;

Photophobia — sunning.

Try to budget half an hour each day for your practice; three-quarters would be better, or you can spend longer if you wish.

The session can be split into two if this is more convenient. Needless to say, glasses should not be worn when practising any of the techniques.

The daily session is used for all those techniques which require either peace and quiet or some item of equipment. Unless you are one of the rare people who have trouble with it, palming should form the basis of your sessions: alternate periods of palming with practice of the other techniques. Aim to practise only those that you enjoy, or that seem specially relevant to your problem. Keep the programme varied so that you do not become bored, and remember to review regularly the techniques you initially rejected to see whether any can after all be incorporated into your schedule.

The eyes work as a dual organ and normally should be treated as such. If one eye is significantly worse than the other, however, and you suspect that it is being "carried" by the stronger eye, then cover the stronger eye with a patch and give the weaker one extra practice of the mobility and accommodation techniques.

Although it is recommended that time should be set aside for practice, awareness of the method must not be restricted to the daily sessions. Take advantage of any spare moment for a little palming or sunning, or for practice in shifting, edging, flashing, and so on. Carry also with you an awareness of the need to blink and breathe easily and freely.

The idea is to improve the use of the eyes, to replace bad habits with good ones. For this to happen the bad habits, acquired perhaps over a period of many years, must be consciously broken and the unconscious habits of good vision with which most of us start out must be actively learned and incorporated into everyday life.

An improvement in use will reduce one source of the strain that leads to refractive error, for "trying" to see will become much less frequent. Reduction of the other source, emotional disturbance, is not so simple. It may well be that your refractive error was caused by some crisis that has been and gone, and that, had you not worn glasses, your eyesight might already have returned to normal. On the other hand, it may be that your refractive error is merely a symptom — perhaps one of several — of some continuing problem. Whatever that may be, and whatever steps you may decide to take in finding a solution, visual re-education is likely to be of some help at least. Just as a negative mental state can affect the eyesight for the worse, so an improvement in eyesight can bring about an improvement in mental outlook. The direction of the vicious circle can be reversed; every small advance made in your Bates training will prepare the way for more and greater advances.

If you have not already given thought to other aspects of the use of your body (as well as to diet, exercise habits, and so on), this might be a good time to do so. It may be appropriate to mention here the Alexander Technique, which is a means of learning and maintaining correct use of the entire organism. Exponents of the technique frequently find that, parallel with improvements in such outwardly obvious aspects of well-being as posture, poise, and the ability to relax, there are corresponding inner improvements. An easy introduction to the subject is given by Michael Gelb in *Body Learning* (Aurum Press, London and New York, 1981). Teachers may be contacted through the Society of Teachers of the Alexander Technique, in London; the North American Society for the Alexander Technique, in New York; and the Australian Society of Teachers of the Alexander Technique (AUSTAT), in Sydney.

Results

It is impossible to say how quickly success will come, if indeed it comes at all. Erring on the side of caution, you should think in terms of one year at least and probably two. Nor is it possible to predict whether you will eventually be able to do without glasses altogether. The worse your eyesight now, and the longer (in years) and the more persistently (each day) you have worn your glasses, the harder it is likely to be. Much of course depends on your own motivation and self discipline. The rate of progress also varies with the individual. Some people, even with quite bad eyesight, respond quickly, while others with only minor problems are not so lucky and must be more patient.

Broadly speaking, the first results come within a few hours or days of starting, but these are so elusive that they are liable to be discounted. Your eyes will probably feel more comfortable and you may find that you are able to distinguish slightly more of the test chart.

This slow, unremarkable progress may turn out to be the general pattern, but, for most people, there will sooner or later (usually within a couple of months) come more convincing evidence. While practising with the test material, or perhaps at some other time, you may experience a brief flash of vision which, if not actually perfect, will be so much better than your usual standard that you will hardly be able to believe your own eyes. This flash will be the first of many, gradually increasing in clarity, frequency, and duration as you proceed. At the same time the quality of your other, "non-flash" vision will be improving.

Your progress may be smoothly continuous, or it may run in steps. In the latter case, progress will be very slow or even absent for several weeks, whereupon there will be a sudden advance. The eyesight then remains more or less static for another period of weeks before the next advance.

In either case, the object of the method is to reach the point where your "non-flash" vision is not greatly inferior to that experienced during flashes. Flash vision is the best that you are currently capable of; non-flash vision is being impaired by the influences that the Bates method sets out to minimise. Since it is not possible to eliminate these influences altogether, you should not imagine that, at some future time, your eyesight will be continuously perfect. It may achieve a very high average standard indeed, but the performance of the eyesight, like that of any human function, is influenced by such variable factors as mood, fatigue, and general state of health.

The method and children

The Bates method is suitable for everyone but the very young. In the first few years of life the skills of binocular and foveal vision must be learned and the appropriate pathways laid down in the brain. In order for that to happen the optical axes must be correctly aligned, and it is most important to have your child's eyes examined no later than the age of three to make sure that all is well. If the necessary skills have not been acquired by the age of six or seven the fault can never be remedied, for by then it is too late to establish the pathways in the brain. Any glasses prescribed before the age of seven should be worn exactly as directed. After this time, however, a child can benefit from the method in just the same way as an adult.

Children are often very responsive to the Bates method,

especially if it is presented in an entertaining way. They usually like to have the letters on the test chart pointed to for them to read; and the more experience of the method you have yourself the better, so that you can not only teach from a position of knowledge but also adapt the various techniques to the child's needs and interests. Right from the very start parents should set a good example with their own visual habits, which, like all other aspects of behaviour, are closely copied by the child.

Many children's games are excellent for the eyesight. "I Spy" is an example; so is the game in which parent and child take it in turns to draw, line by line, some object in the room or visible outdoors which the other has to guess. Car journeys can be enlivened with numberplate games — making words or phrases from the letters, say, or finding particular sequences or combinations. Children are naturally observant and love to exercise their powers of vision, and this should always be given full encouragement by adults.

A personal account

When I started my own Bates training I had no guidance except Bates's book, and knew no one who had achieved any success with the method. It would have been of enormous help to me to have seen a record of someone else's progress and I am including an account of my own, not because it is of any intrinsic interest, but so that you may have something to compare with your own experience.

As a small boy I had excellent eyesight. By the age of 17, though, at a time when I was working hard to qualify for university entrance, and when my studies were in the charge of a master in whom I had but little confidence, I developed very mild myopia in both eyes and was given a pair of glasses. These I wore only when I needed especially sharp vision — for seeing the blackboard, while watching television or at the cinema, and while driving at night. On average I suppose I wore my glasses for an hour or two every day. I kept this same pair for nearly 12 years, during which period I had no eye test: my eyesight had deteriorated no further and was more than adequate for everyday purposes.

At the age of 28, however, during a difficult period in my career, there came an emotional crisis in the form of an acutely unhappy affair; shortly thereafter I began to notice that my old glasses were no longer adequate, and I visited an optician, who prescribed a pair that was very much stronger.

The new glasses were so uncomfortable that I returned to him and asked to have the prescription checked and the test repeated. He assured me that both had been correct and that I would have to learn to get used to the new glasses. I faithfully tried to do so and, although I could never wear them for longer than a couple of hours before developing a headache, I kept this pair for almost two years before going to another optician. This man, while not accepting that his colleague had prescribed glasses that were too strong, nonetheless gave me a pair which was a good deal weaker. The new pair, however, had correction for astigmatism as well as myopia, which the others had not. At that time my vision was about 12:20 in either eye (see Appendix A for the method of measuring visual acuity).

Four months later I happened to notice a copy of *Better Eyesight Without Glasses* in a bookstore. Despite an immediate scepticism, I picked it up out of curiosity and, since I was concerned about the state of my eyesight and was willing to try anything to improve it, I decided, against my better judgement, to buy the book.

My scepticism remained firmly intact as I read it, but, because the practices described seemed harmless enough and there was nothing to lose, I tried some of them out anyway.

On 10 January, the day I bought the book, I put my glasses aside. On 13 January I palmed for a total of 10 minutes. The next day I did the same, and found to my utter amazement and consternation that, after palming, the test chart had become momentarily and marginally easier to read. This was a scientific impossibility, sheer heresy!

Each day I palmed for a total of 10 or 15 minutes and practised shifting with the test chart provided. By 17 January my best vision had improved from 12:20 (60 per cent of normal) to 12:15 (80 per cent). I began to notice that my eyesight seemed clearer and more relaxed generally, both indoors and out. On 27 January I recorded an optimum acuity of 120 per cent, although this lasted only a moment. During the first week of February there came a more marked improvement, and I measured my acuity at 120 per cent several times. My refractive error seemed to be resolving itself into two distinct components. First there was simple myopia, the kind of short-sightedness I had developed at school, in which I was reluctant to look into the distance and everything there seemed uniformly blurred. Then, overlying the simple myopia, was myopic astigmatism, which affected only my distance vision and made vertical lines more blurred than horizontal ones. The first component, the simple myopia, seemed to be responding much more quickly than the astigmatism.

On 7 February I wrote in my notebook:

After palming twice [for 5 minutes at a stretch, and with the test chart 12 feet away] the whole of the bottom of the chart came out quite distinctly for the first time. The 10' and 15' lines were clear and solid black; I felt as if I could have read the 10' line at 20'. This clarity lasted perhaps for 3 seconds — long enough to be appreciable . . . The third palming produced no such clear result.

My next note came on 27 February:

Since making the last entry I have been palming every day for 2, 3, or 4 × 5 minutes, then looking at the chart and sometimes shifting. There has been a consistent improvement in my eyesight; on sunny days in particular, outdoors, I can see such things as the pointing on distant brickwork, twigs high in a tree, etc. I am noticing features of the district which I never knew were there — unusual roof-tiles, leaded windows which I previously thought were of plain glass, and I am seeing and reading notices, signs and lettering of all kinds . . . Today, after palming, my eyes were 20:20, and probably slightly better, for an appreciable time. When they revert to the "pre-palming" state I can distinguish 12:15 without difficulty and a greater or lesser portion of 12:10 — representing vision of about 85–95%. This has been achieved since 13 January; on that day I measured my vision as 60%. Thus, taking the lowest figure now (85%), there has been a 40% improvement since then.

   23 March. For the past four weeks I have been continuing to palm daily and use the test chart. My general vision has slowly improved, and, especially out-of-doors and when the sun shines, I see well at the distance. Four or five days ago the frequency of "clear" flashes when using the chart began to increase — once, then twice each session. About 20–21 March I began, besides palming and shifting, to use the technique described by Bates as "flashing". Almost immediately the clear flashes began coming regularly, among a whole series of minor distortions and of the usual faintly blurred, astigmatic images. Yesterday I found that by blinking I could induce clear flashes — lasting only as long as my lids remained open (i.e., before the next blink) — almost at will. Last night I managed to do this, reading clearly the gilt lettering on the spine of my French dictionary while standing on the opposite side of the room, so well that I felt as if I had entered new territory — passed some important and crucial stage on the way to recovering my vision. This morning on rising I was able to "blink" again. The whole garden, the entire view from my window, was brought for a moment into perfect focus. The colours — of the grass, the distant daffodils, everything — were incredibly fresh, vibrant, rich, yet also wonderfully subtle and soft. Each detail of the wrought iron gate [40 metres (45 yards) away] became, in that instant, a model of clarity. No; not a model — the gate was itself, nothing more or less. I had seen it as if for the first time. The world had become a new and marvellous place. I closed my lids, reopened them, and the familiar, blurred, second-rate version returned.

At this date my eyesight at reading distance, which I had previously imagined to be good, also improved dramatically: I was able to perceive extremely fine detail, and my near point was at about 10 centimetres (4 inches). Plainly, 10 weeks or so of palming and shifting had finally brought about a sudden improvement in my scanning action. A few days later I measured my acuity during a clear flash as 12:6 — twice the normal standard.

So intrigued and excited was I by all this that I read whatever I could about the Bates method and the human visual system, in an effort to find out what was happening. I found that the teachers who had come after Dr Bates had refined his techniques and developed new ones, some of which I introduced to my own practice: domino drills, analytical observation, and various sorts of fusion. Palming, however, with and without visualisation, together with outdoor sunning and use of the test chart for shifting, swinging, and accommodation, remained essential to my daily sessions.

I had developed, soon after being given my strong pair of glasses, a chalazion (a kind of cyst) inside my lower left eyelid. An operation to remove it at the local eye clinic was a failure, as was another performed by a surgeon I went to see privately. The chalazion remained, and I was advised by the second optician that it would eventually need to be removed surgically.

Within two months of starting my Bates training, the chalazion had shrunk to nothing, leaving only the scar tissue from the operations and a redness inside the eyelid. The redness too subsequently went. Except for the very slight thickening caused by the scar tissue, the eyelid now appears perfectly normal.

My eyesight continued to improve fairly steadily. The clear flashes began coming with greater frequency, but, more importantly, my non-flash vision was improving also. A year after starting, my simple myopia had virtually disappeared. The myopic astigmatism was the main cause of imperfection. I could see horizontal objects clearly into the farthest distance, but still had a little trouble with vertical ones, except during clear flashes, when my vision was perfect. A year after that the gap between my flash and non-flash vision had closed still more, and it still continues to close. My non-flash vision now never seems to drop below about 85 per cent, and is usually considerably better than that. At the age of 35 my nearpoint remains at 10 centimetres (4 inches) and my ability to perceive detail is, if anything, increasing.

I feel that the worst damage was done to my vision by the overstrong glasses I was prescribed. Had it not been for those — had I learned about the Bates method when still wearing my first pair — I doubt that my recovery would have taken so long. On the other hand, I count myself fortunate indeed that I was not in the habit of wearing my glasses continuously, that I was able to do without them from the first day, that I was comparatively young when I started, and that my problem was so mild to begin with.

In conclusion

An individual's Bates training is rather like a voyage of discovery. The final goal will probably be rather different from the one imagined at the outset. Before embarking, however, it helps to have some idea at least of what one is hoping to achieve. "Freedom from glasses" is the short answer, but what does that imply?

The practical disadvantages of glasses are many and various and need not be listed here. Of more concern are the effects, in the long term as well as the short, that glasses have on vision.

Each air-to-glass surface reduces the transmission of light and alters the perception of colour. Everything seems much harsher when viewed through glass or plastic. The image is further degraded by the difficulty of keeping the lenses clean.

Whether their lenses are concave or convex, glasses alter the apparent size of objects and seriously cut down the field of view, both by physical obstruction and by preventing free rotation of the eyes in the head, for one must look through the optical centres of the lenses in order to see clearly. This in turn leads to problems. Compared with the engineering of the eye, spectacle frames are of decidedly inferior construction. They are far too clumsy to allow any but an approximate alignment of the optical centres of the lenses with the optical axes; and, even if the best possible alignment is achieved when the glasses are first fitted, ordinary wear and tear soon knocks them out of true — to the detriment of the functioning of the eye.

Most of these effects can be mitigated by using contact lenses, but contact lenses share with glasses the most serious disadvantage of all: the perpetuation of refractive error.

If it is accepted that the eye does indeed change shape during accommodation, and that the eye has evolved to work in the absence of refractive error (that is, that the eye should shorten and lengthen only within fairly narrow limits), it follows that an eye with refractive error, especially an error which is being perpetuated by the use of glasses, is being subjected to continuous distortion.

The blood supply inside the eye and the drainage of excess intraocular fluid depend on the free operation of exceedingly fine vessels and channels. As much as the eye is distorted, these will tend to be restricted. If the supply of nourishment and the removal of waste are impeded, the health of the tissues is bound to decline and ageing processes such as hardening of the lens are likely to progress more rapidly. If the drainage of the eye is impeded, there may well be an increase in intraocular pressure, of just the kind associated with the condition known as chronic simple glaucoma.

Thus, if the Bates hypothesis is correct, glasses and contact lenses are not only a nuisance, but also represent a potential threat to the long-term health of the eye. For this reason the Bates method can be looked upon as a form of preventive medicine.

Beyond the purely practical benefits of going without glasses lie others, less obvious, but real enough all the same. The eyesight is one of our two most important senses. Through it we gather much of our knowledge of the world. To interpose an artificial barrier between our eyes and our environment represents a fundamental interference with the natural process of perception. If our perception is faulty, so too in equal measure will be our whole attitude to life, our behaviour, and our beliefs.

As the vision slowly improves, one finds one's personality subtly changing — or rather, one finds some of its hidden potential being realised — in the direction of balance, reason, and independence. In the later stages of the Bates training such considerations as these can become even more rewarding than the unalloyed and life-enhancing pleasure of better eyesight.

APPENDIX A

Measuring Visual Acuity

The optician's test chart was devised by the Dutch ophthalmologist Hermann Snellen (1835–1908). In its usual form it consists of a number of lines of letters of decreasing size. Each line is assigned a distance at which it should be legible to the normal eye; the eyesight is considered normal if the six-metre line can indeed be read at six metres. This standard is expressed as a fraction, or a ratio, so that normal vision is described as 6/6, or 6:6. Someone with only half this acuity would be described as having 3:6 vision; someone with only a third 2:6, and so on. At one time the distance was measured in feet, and 20:20 is the same standard as 6:6.

The distance at which the chart is read is that at which the height of the letter subtends an angle of five minutes of arc (see Figure 12). This value has been chosen quite arbitrarily and in fact represents only a rather mediocre standard of acuity. A standard of 12:6 is regularly attained by people with good eyesight.

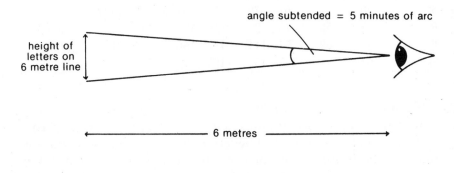

Figure 12 (not to scale)

ACUITY TABLES FOR USE WITH TEST CHARTS
1 Metric units

Chart C at 25	37.5	50	62.5	75	87.5	100	112.5	125	cm
Chart B at 50	75	100	125	150	175	200	225	250	cm
Chart A at 2	3	4	5	6	7	8	9	10	m
C (60 m)	3	5	7	8	10	12	13	15	17	%
E (36 m)	6	9	11	14	17	19	22	25	28	
O (24 m)	8	13	17	21	25	29	33	38	42	
D (18 m)	11	17	22	28	33	39	44	50	56	
U (12 m)	17	25	33	42	50	58	67	75	83	
F (9 m)	22	33	44	56	67	78	89	100	111	
S (6 m)	33	50	67	83	100	117	133	150	167	
R (5 m)	40	60	80	100	120	140	160	180	200	
B (4 m)	50	75	100	125	150	175	200	(225)	(250)	
H (3 m)	67	100	133	167	200	(233)	(267)	(300)	(333)	

2 Imperial units

Chart C at 9	13.5	18	22.5	27	31.5	36	40.5	45	in
Chart B at 18	27	36	45	54	63	72	81	90	in
Chart A at 6	9	12	15	18	21	24	27	30	ft
C	3	5	6	8	9	11	12	14	15	%
E	5	8	10	13	15	18	20	23	25	
O	8	11	15	19	23	27	30	34	38	
D	10	15	20	25	30	36	41	46	51	
U	15	23	30	38	45	53	61	69	76	
F	20	31	41	51	61	71	81	91	102	
S	30	46	61	76	91	107	122	137	152	
R	37	55	73	91	110	128	146	165	183	
B	46	69	91	114	137	160	183	(206)	(229)	
H	61	91	122	152	183	(213)	(244)	(274)	(305)	

To measure your own visual acuity, fix the large test chart (Chart A) at a distance of four to eight metres (four to nine yards) and in a good strong light. The letters have been chosen with the Bates method rather than the standard specification in mind, but generally the chart conforms to the standard and will give an accurate result when used with care.

With either eye singly, and then with both together, record the lowest line on which you can read all the letters. Then, knowing how far away the chart is, use the Acuity Table to find your acuity. In the table acuity has been expressed as a percentage rather than a ratio. Thus 6:6 is expressed as 100 per cent, 9:6 as 150 per cent, etc. As an example, if on Chart A you can read the whole of the 9-metre line (the one beginning with the letter F) at a maximum distance of 7 metres, your acuity works out at 78 per cent of normal.

The table may also be used to find your acuity at reading distance. If at 50 centimetres you can read the whole of the "H" line on Chart C, your acuity is 133 per cent of normal. For convenience the table is also given in imperial units.

As mentioned above, the Snellen standard has been chosen quite arbitrarily. A measure of absolute acuity, finding the smallest object that can be perceived, is in some ways preferable. Each cone in the centre of the foveola covers an area of the visual field which subtends an angle of less than 20 seconds of arc. (There are 60 seconds in one minute of arc, and 3600 seconds in one degree.) With the foveola stationary (that is, not taking the scanning action into account), one should in theory be able, at a range of 1.6 kilometres (1 mile), to perceive an object 15 centimetres (6 inches) across. After Bates training, resolution of 10 seconds of arc or better, representing, at 1.6 kilometres (1 mile), an object some 7.5 centimetres (3 inches) across, is readily achievable. The final limit depends on the refinement and quality of the individual's visual system.

Absolute acuity, measured in seconds of arc ("), may be calculated according to the formula:

$$\text{acuity} = \frac{\text{width of object perceived} \times 206265,}{\text{range}}$$

assuming that both measurements are in the same units. If range is measured in metres and width in millimetres, divide by 1000, so that the formula becomes:

$$\text{acuity} = \frac{\text{width} \times 206}{\text{range}}$$

If range is measured in yards and width in inches, the formula is:

$$\text{acuity} = \frac{\text{width} \times 5730}{\text{range}}$$

Thus if you can discern a power line 100 millimetres in diameter at a range of 3 kilometres (3000 metres), your absolute acuity works out at $\frac{100 \times 206}{3000}$, or 7″ (7 seconds of arc).

Acuity is of course improved in conditions of good lighting, contrast, and clarity of air. Any object at any range may be used for this test, but, due to the scanning action of the eye, single objects (flagpoles, golfballs, etc.) are not so rapidly perceived as multiple ones. A grid of lines makes a more suitable datum for an acuity test. The pointing in brickwork, particularly if it contrasts well with the colour of the bricks, is ideal. For example, if the average width of the pointing on a wall is 10 millimetres, and you can perceive the pointing at a maximum range of 125 metres, your absolute acuity is $\frac{10 \times 206}{125}$, or 16″.

APPENDIX B

Visual Material

Random number table
Sight-testing Chart A (inside front cover)
Charts B and C
Chart D (inside back cover)
Astigmatism indicator

RANDOM NUMBER TABLE

32	97	34	18	23	73	98	68	03	03
17	81	36	95	27	82	98	22	65	32
82	68	35	79	32	54	44	39	94	98
17	71	10	34	74	52	82	07	12	68
50	66	38	88	51	83	52	15	13	01
11	08	29	52	25	86	11	37	59	87
12	36	64	79	22	80	82	61	64	82
08	05	89	98	73	51	97	87	26	36
24	48	63	83	15	53	34	54	47	78
30	61	23	90	87	13	20	91	56	54
62	87	44	77	16	39	67	20	98	19
57	84	38	86	61	51	89	80	88	87
16	65	72	54	70	35	29	82	85	01
48	34	91	49	27	94	14	89	42	45
11	36	53	10	42	22	59	29	35	89
71	37	22	33	89	29	66	34	20	22
79	53	54	39	24	81	91	05	67	78
33	21	27	31	74	76	69	24	05	68
50	86	43	83	39	90	74	93	04	43
03	03	49	53	22	30	82	01	85	28
55	46	67	53	34	63	93	31	14	87
22	05	82	03	90	16	03	39	24	98
39	58	77	51	32	87	47	41	41	75
23	84	59	54	57	55	51	21	62	92
20	71	11	73	37	06	44	55	31	04
36	91	43	91	03	29	02	39	26	48
35	87	10	51	54	60	97	12	76	54
44	46	40	85	69	32	72	23	30	06
83	57	12	84	38	96	08	11	54	53
05	21	11	51	43	27	23	70	84	96
78	33	59	71	09	56	78	66	84	20
20	47	10	33	99	35	89	82	13	89
82	84	12	74	13	54	29	77	62	05
50	68	87	61	67	80	34 ·	77	69	18
47	01	19	56	35	61	12	23	77	91

CHART B

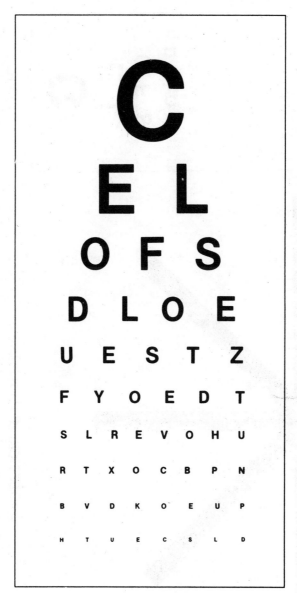

C
E L
O F S
D L O E
U E S T Z
F Y O E D T
S L R E V O H U
R T X O C B P N
B V D K O E U P
H T U E C S L D

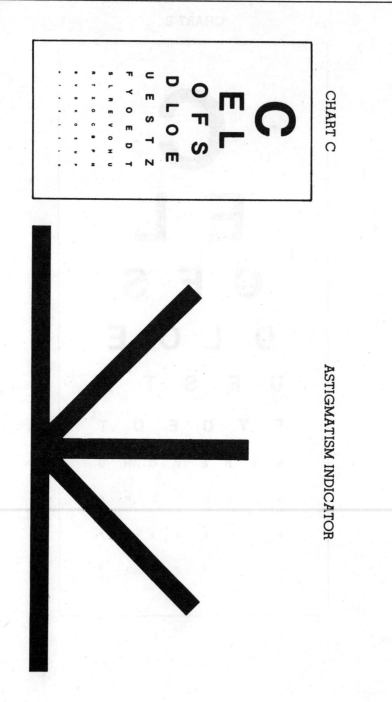

CHART C

ASTIGMATISM INDICATOR

Index